50 INVALUABLE LIFE-LESSONS I'VE LEARNED IN 50 YEARS!

(General Readership)

50 INVALUABLE LIFE-LESSONS I'VE LEARNED IN 50 YEARS!

(General Readership)

By

Dr. Sammy O. Joseph

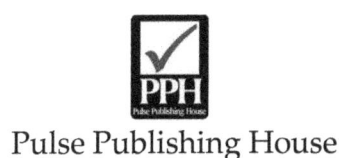

Pulse Publishing House

© 2019 Sammy O. Joseph

Published in the United Kingdom by
Pulse Publishing House
Box 15129
Birmingham
England B45 5DJ
publishinghouse@harvestways.org

All rights reserved. No part of this publication may be reproduced, stored in a retrieval system, or be transmitted, in any form, or by any means, mechanical, electronic, photocopying or otherwise without the prior written consent of the publisher.

Bible quotes are from the King James Version of the Bible unless otherwise stated.

Amplified quotes are from the Amplified Bible, © copyright 1995 by The Zondervan Corporation and The Lockman Foundation.

Cover design and typesetting by Pulse Publishing House, England.

ISBN 978-0-9567298-6-6

Contents

Dedication   *xi*

Quick Word   *xii*

Book 1: Giving   1

  #1: Never Forget to Treat Yourself to the Best Gifts Too!   3

  #2: Give Not your Gifts to Dogs nor Cast your Pearls before the Swine!   5

  #3: Feed Healthy foods only to Your Stomach.   7

  #4: Give respect. Expect Respect.   8

  #5: Be Deliberate upon Delivering that which You Conceived!   10

  #6: You're Responsible for Your Harvests.   12

  #7: Smear Some on You too!   14

  #8: Give Yourself a Fairer Chance Than You Gave to Others.   16

  #9: Give no Power to Any to De-humanize You.   18

  #10: "Vox Populi, Vox Dei!"   20

Book 2: Family, Ministry, Business & Corporate Matters — 23

#11: False Humility will Limit You! — *25*

#12: Prioritize Family Above Ministry/Business Organization. — *27*

#13: Involve Your Family in the Ministry/Business Organization. — *29*

#14: Differentiate Roles in the Family, Ministry/Business. — *32*

#15: Specialize in Your Core; Be it Family, Ministry/Business. — *34*

#16: Don't let a Crushing Cause You an Offense against Christ Jesus. — *37*

#17: If God promised it, He will Deliver it! Trust Him through – and thoroughly! — *40*

#18: Be Ruthless with Weeds Generally wherever They're found; Either in a Family, Ministry/Business. — *43*

#19: Handling a Prodigal's Return to the Fold. — *45*

#20: Understanding Mirages in the Family, Ministry/Business. — *47*

Book 3: Listening for Divine Instructions in Wisdom on Cogent Matters — 49

#21: Wrathful Fight with God on specific instructions

Relating to Family, Ministry/Business.	*51*
#22: When You've Been Lifted High by God, Never Forget Your Roots!	*54*
Book 4: Friends Contrasted with Fiends	57
#23: Contrasting the word "Friend" with "Fiends."	*59*
#24: "F" stands for "Fierce Loyalty."	*61*
#25: "R" stands for "Ruthlessness in Attracting – and Keeping Friends!"	*64*
#26: "I" stands for "Intricate interest."	*66*
#27: "E" stands for "Expectation of a high Yield of Returns!"	*69*
#28: "N" stands for "Never become Nebulous in a Friendship."	*72*
#29: "D" stands for "Dependability in Friendship."	*75*
#30: "S" stands for "Sensitivity in Friendship."	*77*
#31: Boundaries & Confrontations in Friendship.	*80*
#32: 'Kitty-Katty' Friends!	*83*
Book 5: Single, Engaged, Married, Sex and Sexuality	87
#33: Complete Singleness.	*89*

#34: Be intently Focused on Hearing from God by Yourself. — 92

#35: When She is Genuinely interested in You! — 95

#36: When He is Genuinely interested in You! — 98

#37: Never Get Engaged without first Learning how to Harmoniously Resolve Your Disagreements! — 101

#38: Getting Engaged? Never "Cut off" Your Parent(s). — 104

#39: Wedding/Marriage Preparations. — 108

#40: Marriage! — 110

#41: The Gift of Sex and Sexuality. — 112

Book 6: Unhealthy Marriage, Separation & Divorce – and Co-Habitation — 115

#42: Unhealthy Marriage, Counseling, Separation, Divorce – and Cohabitation. — 117

#43: Cohabiting Ex-spouses. — 120

#44: Life after Divorce. — 124

Book 7: Raising Godly Children — 129

#45: Show God to Your Children Early in Life. — 131

#46: Always Apply the 'Fair-play' Rule to the Child. — 134

#47: Money-matter and Strong Work Ethics. — 137

#48: When Children Leave Home.	139
Book 8: Healthy Foods/Drink Choices	**143**
# 49: Eat Greaseless, Healthy Meals!	145
#50: Drink Healthy, Costless, Home-made Drinks.	147
Book 9: Extras on Health & Fitness; and Healthy Lifestyle Choices	**149**
#1: The Best Healthy Food of All Times: The Bible.	151
#2: Eat Healthy, Home-cooked foods.	152
#3: Eat Bitter Melons.	154
#4: Snack on Dried Nuts.	155
#5: Say 'No' to Donuts.	157
#6: A Word of Caution on Red-meat.	158
#7: A Word of Caution on Processed food, Generally.	159
#8. Mental Awareness Needs.	160
#9. 'Gymnos' Acknowledgment.	165
#10. The Appropriate Use of a Gymnasium – Or other Health & Fitness Facilities.	167
10. A Closing Remark	**171**

Dedication

This project in your hands is somewhat personal to me. It is dedicated it to my spiritual father, Dr. Creflo Dollar who has nurtured and sustained my spirit and soul – for a period of over two decades – in *that* famished season of life others had simply vanished out of!

Quick Word

When you turn fifty, you want to do something radical. Something you've never done in your entire livelihood. Some folk will go skydiving in the atmosphere with the birds. Others, scuba-diving in the oceans with the sharks – and other sea creatures. Some brave hearts will go on a sabbatical holiday to some faraway lands. Well, I haven't done any of those, at least not yet. Instead, Father-God inspired me yet this tenth time to sit down – and write. (Achieving ten published works in eight years isn't a bad feat for one who felt God's Spirit challenged them to produce a thousand volumes before they are recalled Home!)

So, this volume is excitingly different to all others before it. In it, I have made disclosures about myself, my immediate family and ministry that I had never – in any of my writings or sermons – hitherto revealed!

With the help of my able assistant, Gabby Joseph – when she had arrived home for a brief holiday – I have conscientiously gathered and arranged for you; life, wisdom-nuggets I had gained over the period specified. These lessons, I believe, will help transform and very possibly navigate you through life's meandering courses. I hope this volume becomes one of your *"Delightful books!"*

All the carefully-picked topics of discussion have an urgency about them. They also have pictures in black and white - with italicized, quotable, highlighted quotes from each lesson!

Once you're convinced that you're hungry for an unparalleled truth, search no further. Here's your quick wisdom book. I have discussed briefly but succinctly, topics harsh-tagged such as: *#Invaluable #Lessons #In #Fifty #Years #Talking #About #Gifts #Ministry #Family #Finances #Integrity #Priority #Finding #Your #Passion #Mirages #Emotions #Genuine #Friends #Friendship #Singleness #Marriage #Separation #Divorce #Cohabitation #LifeafterDivorce #Loneliness #Sensitivity #Boundaries #Confrontation #Giving #Healthy #FoodChoices #Foods #Longevity #IncreasedLifeSpan #ChildRaising #ChildBearing #Wise #Choices #Health #Is #Wealth #DontGambleYourHealthAway #FoodsThatHeal #HealthyLifestyle #Exercise #MentalAwareness #MentalHealth #Eat #Drink* and *#Wellness*.

May this piece of writing tremendously bless you!

Sammy Joseph
Birmingham,
England,
January 2019.

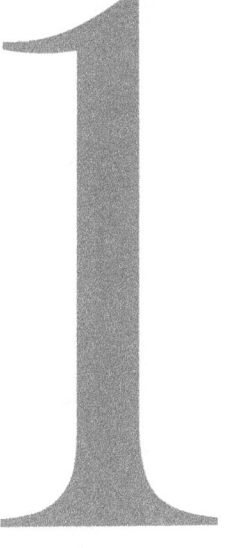

Part One

Giving

Lesson #1: Never Forget to Treat Yourself to the Best Gifts Too!

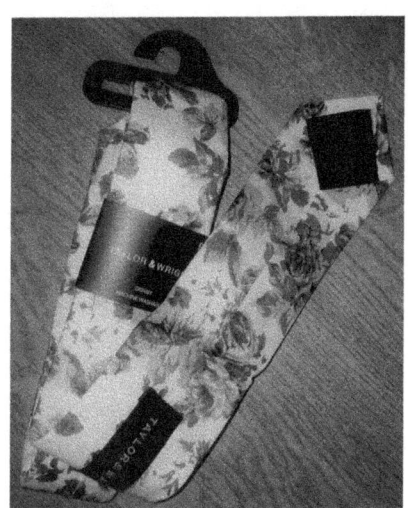

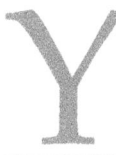

You must possess an excellent spirit to transform 'losses' into 'wins'. One of the ways you achieve that feat is by *giving to yourself, timely, relevant gifts – better than you give to others*. Such gifts as "me-time", occasional treats, travel to destinations longed-for, ticking activities off your bucket-list; cars, fancy clothes, jewelry, houses and such the like.

There's never a period of time that I had forgotten to treat myself to occasional, pretty, beautiful dressing ties and hankie-sets; a bespoke suit, and/or a pair of shoes. That just happens to be an example of my self-reward, to me after I had experienced a win – or a pain!

Value you!

Say often to you: "You're loved!"

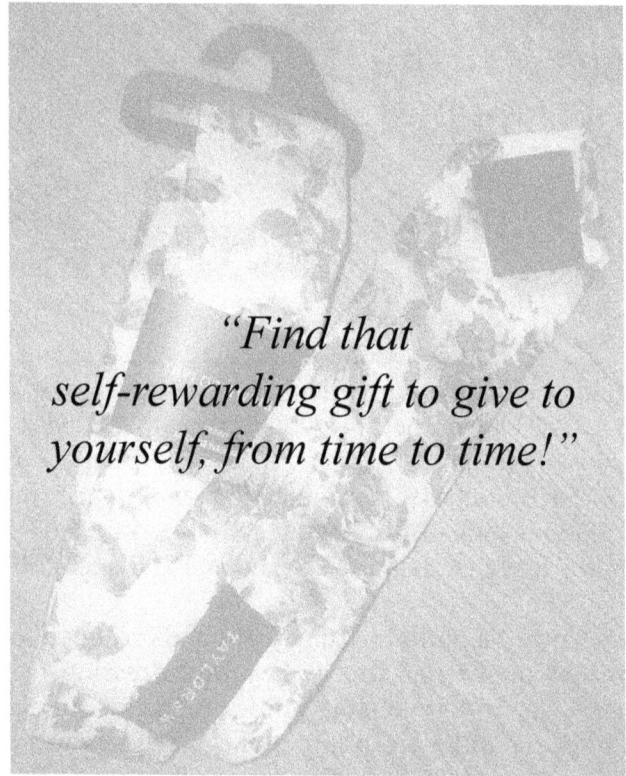

"Find that self-rewarding gift to give to yourself, from time to time!"

The original photograph on the preceding page shows a flowery, skinny tie; one of the author's necktie collections, courtesy of SJM, Birmingham, England. Copyrights reserved.

Lesson #2: Give Not your Gifts to Dogs nor Cast your Pearls before the Swine!

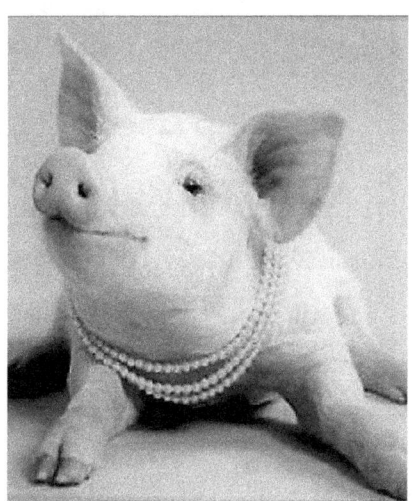

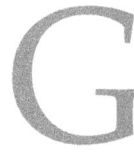

Give *not* your gifts to the dogs, neither cast your pearls before the swine! Jesus Christ warned us against doing that. The Apostles reiterated His teaching – and I eventually learned the principle of *Matthew 7:6* –

> *"Give not that which is holy unto the dogs, neither cast ye your pearls before swine, lest they trample them under their feet, and turn again and rend you."*

There are – at least – three, cogent reasons why the Lord had warned you against making embroidery designs - and wearing them on the dogs and the swine in that Scriptural portion of *Matthew 7:6*. Can you find them?

If you did, name them here, below:

Reason 1:

_____

_____

Reason 2:

_____

_____

Reason 3:

_____

_____

> *"There are – at least – three, cogent reasons why the Lord had warned you against making embroidery designs – and wearing them on the dogs and the swine!"*

Photo credit: The link to the original picture on the preceding page:
http://paperlief.com/pigs/black-piglets-wallpaper-2.html was accessed August 7, 2018, at 23:05hrs.

Lesson #3: Feed Healthy foods only to Your Stomach.

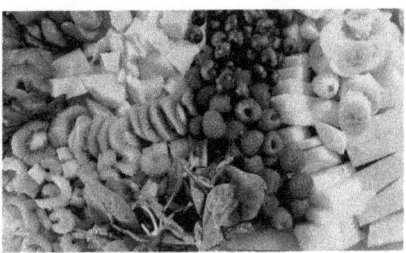

Whatever goes into your stomach eventually builds your tissues, muscles and body's cells. Be careful, therefore, of what you put into your stomach. Feed it only healthy meals and drinks.

In the latter part of this book, I shall hint at healthy and unhealthy foods and drinks.

> *"Remember, you really are what you eat!"*

Photo credit: Gabby Studio, Lancaster, Lancs., England. Copyrights reserved.

Lesson #4: Give Respect; Expect Respect.

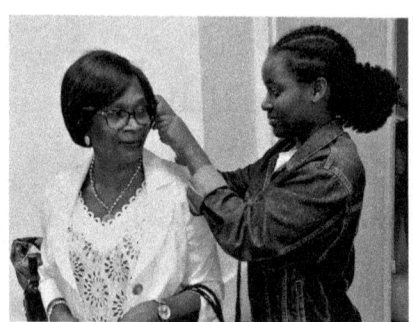

My biological parents were respectable members of the society. They drilled into us – children – from very young ages: *Giving and Expecting Respect!* I did the same for my children – and even, my spiritual children. I always said to them: **"Give respect. Expect respect!"**

I have reproduced below, part of my parents' school of thought to us as we grew up:

- *Dress the way you would love to be addressed.*

- *Speak to others the same way you would love to be spoken to.*

- *Honor others the very same way you would love to be honored, and if your honor is not returned unto you, then:*

- *Respectfully confront them with your expectations!*

Now, I noticed as I grew up that sometimes, hardened narcissistic, controlling, selfish souls are best confronted by their consciences with your peaceful withdrawal from them. That is, your peaceful, walking away without a backward glance!

I had peacefully walked away from abusive, narcissistic, gaslighting individuals many a time – and each time, it had been a win-win for me! Let me encourage you to adapt my style, just for once!

"Hardened narcissistic, controlling, selfish souls are best confronted by their consciences with your peaceful withdrawal!"

The lesson-depicting photograph on the preceding page has been provided courtesy of SJM, Birmingham, England. Copyrights reserved.

Lesson #5:
Be Deliberate upon Delivering that which You Conceived!

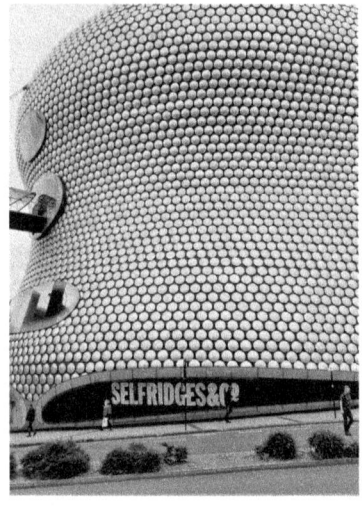

T

This is the side view of the *Selfridges* at Birmingham's *Bullring Shopping Mall*, the largest in Europe. The Bullring itself makes a bespoke statement: No other building in the world has its design! Guess who made that happen?

The architects!

They were deliberate upon delivery: From conception onto the drawing boards, onto its civil engineering calculations of construction material needed – and the very delivery of the goods and materials; the different professionals involved were deliberate, focused, driven and passionate!

Apostle Paul says: *"It is God Who works in you both to will and do of His great pleasure"* | Philippians 2:13.

Giving

As the Father-God works, so you too work. He works purposefully, so you too can work purposefully. His intent is not hidden, so yours too need not be hidden. Be intent and deliberate upon the delivery of the intent you conceived!

Only when you have done that would you have rewarded the world with the gift of intuition the Heavenly Father had endowed you with.

Therefore, be bold to make a bespoke statement on any project you lay your hands upon, from the conception stage to the actualization stage. Don't be afraid to make mistakes. Be focused! There's a huge reward awaiting you upon the completion – and the delivery – of the masterpiece.

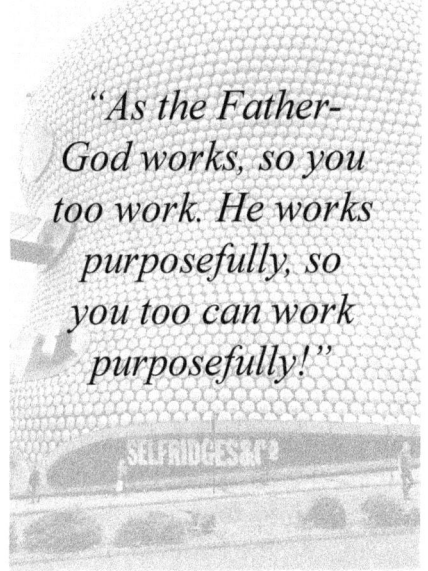

"As the Father-God works, so you too work. He works purposefully, so you too can work purposefully!"

The original photograph on the preceding page reveals the Selfridges, Bullring Shopping Complex, Birmingham, England, courtesy of SJM, Copyrights reserved.

Lesson #6: You're Responsible for Your Harvests.

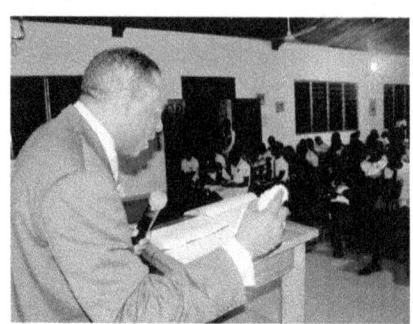

Spiritual farmers are not different from everyday, earthly farmers. If you're an earthly farmer, you wouldn't disagree with this truth: Not every soil yields the hundredfold returns or increase. So, choose carefully the soil into which you plant your seeds – and prioritize your labor of outpouring!

Between sowing and harvesting, lots of activities go on only he the sower can attest unto. Activities like watering the seeds, weeding, mulching, hoeing, staking and training soft, twining tendrils; rebuking worms and building scarecrows to scare the birds off! Finally, the farmer fetches his baskets – and into the fields he goes, reaping the harvest and preserving the fruits in the barns. From these harvests, he will sow again in the next season!

"Not every soil yields the hundredfold returns or increase. So, choose carefully the soil into which you plant your seeds!"

The original photograph on the preceding page shows Dr. Sammy Joseph in a late-night ministration at a Youth Conference in Elmina, Ghana, 2014 courtesy of SJM, Birmingham, England. Copyrighted.

Lesson #7:
Smear Some on You too!

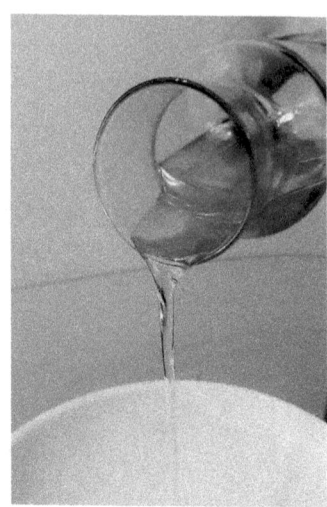

If you're an anointed, outpouring, out-giving soul, the tendency is that you will be tempted of the devil – and by bigoted religious folks to pour all of the oil out on others – and die 'empty'.

You've probably heard it said: *"The anointing is not for you – but for those you've been assigned and sent!"* In some way, that statement may be factual. The only problem is that such a saying will *not* stand the test of the truth! The truth is:

> *It's not a sin to smear some oil on yourself, too!*

You are, after all, *the* assigned jar; the earthen vessel that carries the anointing! Apostle Paul humbly reminds us all: *"We have this treasure in earthen vessels ..."* | *2 Corinthians 4:7.*

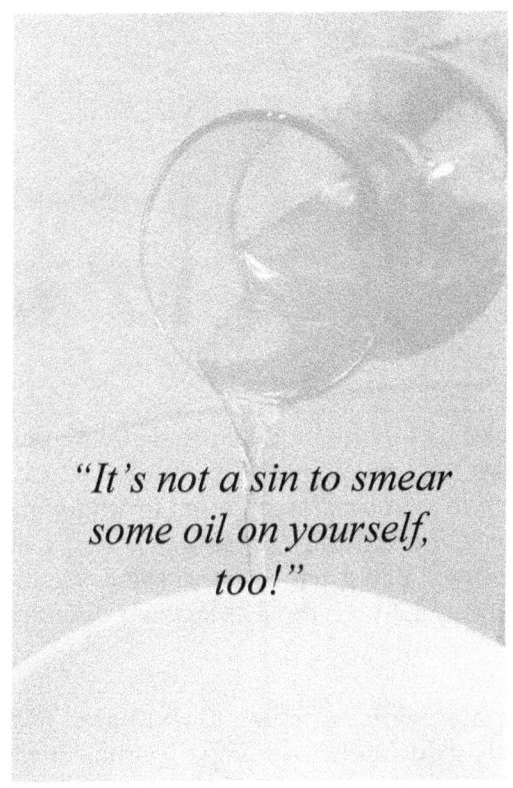

"It's not a sin to smear some oil on yourself, too!"

The original photograph on the preceding page reveals a vial of anointing oil outpoured from a jar.
Copyrighted, SJM.

Lesson #8:
Give Yourself a Fairer Chance Than You Gave to Others.

F

For many years growing up, I struggled with perfectionist traits, ideas, and ideologies. My childhood struggles did *not* emerge from my parents' doing or undoing. Dad and mom were educated minds: He was a soil scientist with the Department of Agriculture and she, a senior management educationist with the Department of Education, until her retirement.

Being the most spiritual of their four children, at a very tender age, I had deviated towards perfectionism: Shoes must be on the shoe-rack in order. Shirts must be displayed on hangers hung in the wardrobes – or neatly folded by their corners, kept away in lockers; pairs of socks kept in pairs, dishes hand-washed, drained, dried, wiped and stored away. Grammarly-speaking, the pronunciation of every syllable in the word was a must – and so on and so forth. Maybe it was a good thing. Maybe not! The only problem was that my 'idealist' thoughts came at a personal cost; the costliest being, self-depersonification!

Self-depersonification makes you become your own worst critic whilst praising others. It ensures that you fail to forgive yourself for life's opportunities missed. Self-depersonification makes you become self-denigrating!

I think, having passed through the twists and the turns on the highways and the low tunnels of life, I am more than qualified to instruct you: Stop severely, unjustly critiquing yourself. Particularly when you fall short of – either people's or your personal – expectations!

Give yourself more than a chance. Celebrate you. Enjoy *your* life: You won't satisfy everyone – and that's okay!

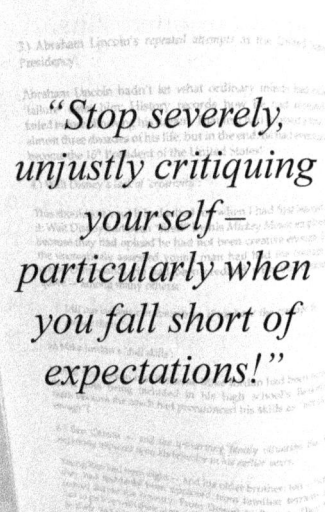

The original screenshot picture shows page 6, 'GIDEON: Releasing the Potentials Within You' by Dr. Sammy O. Joseph, PULSE Publishing House, UK. Revised edition, 2018. Copyrighted.

Lesson #9:
Give no Power to Any to De-humanize You.

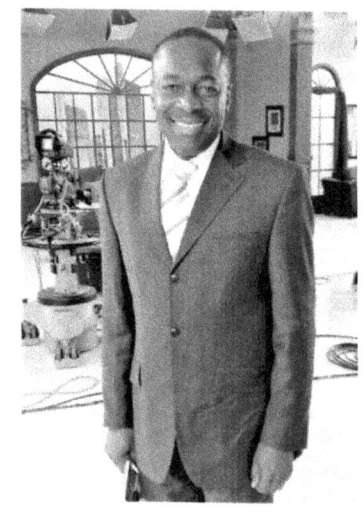

Cameras and images are often illusory. Only what lies within or behind the glares of the lenses is worth the reckon! *Lesson #9* reads: *"Give no power to any to de-humanize you."*

Some people will attempt to de-humanize you by deifying you. Be smart enough to quickly remind them that you are *not* God. You are just an anointed being. Ask them to ask Lucifer! Many others will attempt to disenfranchise you by making you beg for what's rightfully yours. Others some, will try to enslave you.

Remember you are no more your own. You've been bought with – and indeed redeemed at – a price. You now have a better, re-possessed self-worth in Christ Jesus! Protect fiercely, therefore, *your* worth. *Your* inheritance. *Your* territory. Do not entertain compromising situations close to your quarters for any reason! Ignite the power of *your* integrity!

Never give anyone the power to manipulate, de-humanize or enslave *you*.

Never!

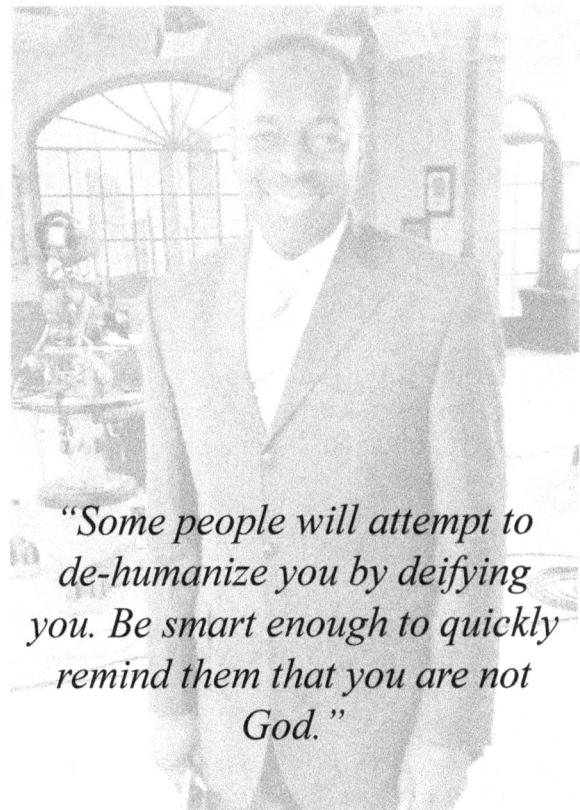

"*Some people will attempt to de-humanize you by deifying you. Be smart enough to quickly remind them that you are not God.*"

The lesson-depicting photo overleaf shows Dr. Sammy Joseph's maiden live-telecast to over 100 million views across the world on 'Celebrate Live' at the former TCT-TV Studio, Southfield, Detroit, Michigan, U.S.A. April 4, 2015. Copyrighted, SJM.

Lesson #10:
Vox Populi, Vox Dei!

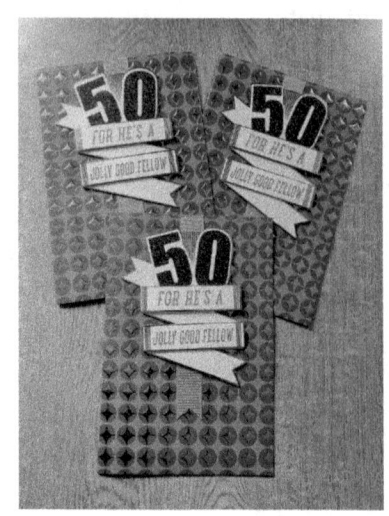

Forgive me for still basking in the glory of the golden number, *fifty*. But I have also learned a reasonable approval rating percentage you should endeavor to maintain as you gracefully grow older.

"What about it?" you asked!

The Holy Bible categorically records our Lord's denunciation of the scoffing *"Pharisees who loved money"* in *Luke 16:14* thus:

> *"You are they which justify yourselves before men; God knows your hearts – for that which is highly esteemed before men is an abomination in the sight of God."*
>
> | *Luke 16:15*

In my indulged state of mind, I dare conjecture, the following as healthy human ratings:

i.) 85% APPROVAL of you;

ii.) 5-7% DISAPPROVAL of you; and

iii.) 8-10% UNDECIDED about you!

Now, if either everyone approves or disapproves of you generally; or you're one who loves to praise him/herself, trust me, *"You're beat!"*

I must have taken a beating upon realizing that three of the few cards given by friends at my half-centennial celebration had been exactly the same – word-verbatim, on the outside, that is! How coincidental, I had thought! Father-God must have a jolly good approval rating of His son down here in Northfield!

Now, the unbeatable truth is that the voices of a holy people are more often, the very voice of God! That was an unforgettable lesson that the Lord would have me take notice of: *"Vox Populi, Vox Dei!"*

"The voices of a holy people are more often, the very voice of God!"

The lesson-depicting photo of cards overleaf was supplied courtesy of Sammy Joseph Ministries. *(Three similar cards given by some Friends of SJM during Dr. Joseph's 50th Birthday celebrations, March 24, 2018; Birmingham, England.)*

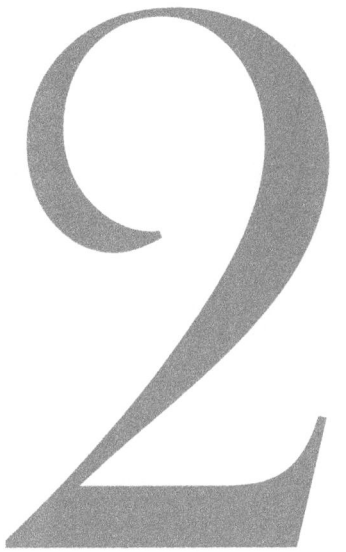

PART TWO

Family,
Ministry,
Business &
Corporate
Matters

Lesson #11: False Humility will Limit You!

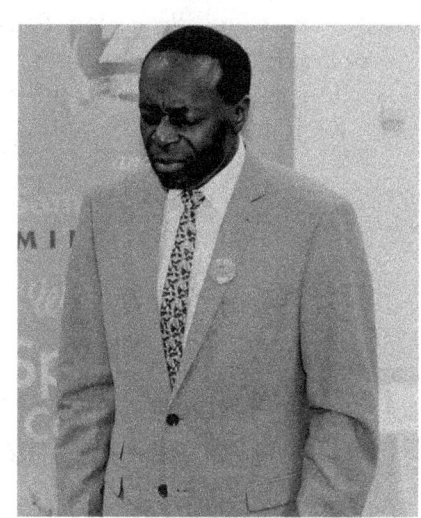

Humility is healthy in every ramification of life's endeavor. Whether it is family, ministry, or business structure! But when you possess a sense of false humility, you begin to rot – and will soon release a pungent smell of total un-healthiness. In fact, false-humility is a biting pride in disguise!

Over a decade ago, a man rang me and said: *"God told me to sow £1000.00 into your ministry!"*

I replied: *"Oh no; please don't do that. We'd be okay with a hundred!"*

And that was the exact amount he had sown! I had only short changed myself. I later felt that the good Lord must have taught me an unforgettable lesson!

In this new decade, however, I honestly believe that I have by now mastered *the* lesson: False humility will limit you, your family, ministry/business. Not only that, it should also limit all that God would have accomplished with – and through you!

Declare aloud with me straightaway: *"Lord, be it unto me, according to Your word!"*

Over a decade ago, a man called me up and said: "God told me to sow £1000.00 into your ministry!"

I replied: "Oh no; please don't do that. We'd be okay with a hundred!"

The original picture on the preceding page shows Dr. Sammy Joseph at the annual Spring Up Conference which takes place the third weekend of every March in Birmingham, England. Photo courtesy SJM, Birmingham, England. Copyrighted.

Lesson #12: Prioritize Family Above Ministry/Business Organization.

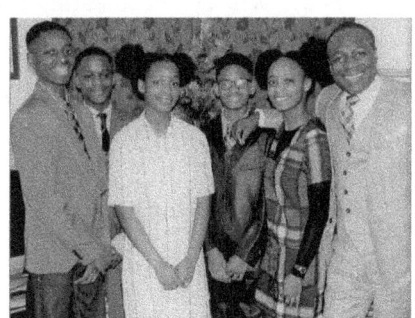

I

If anyone were to ask you: *"Which is your priority – ministry, business, or family? Wealth or a lasting relationship?"* How would you order?

If you were like me, I'd put in a quick order for both. But were I instructed to sever one and keep the other as the necessary option, it must be for me: *Family before ministry – and lasting relationships, well above wealth!*

The rationale influencing my thought pattern is: After everything is said and done, the only ones you would always impact the greatest are your family – and circle of loved ones!

Since eternity, people had always come and gone. Only those who have come to recognize you as their parent will forever be faithful – and loyal to you! This is the reason why you choose them above everything else – after God! This is the wisest ministerial and investment sense!

Do you agree or disagree?

(Write me your opinion as a feedback. Your note will not be shared without first asking for your permission. My addresses are at the back of the book.)

"The only ones you would always impact the greatest are your family – and circle of loved ones!"

The preceding page reveals the photo of the Josephs from their 2016 Christmas family-album. Copyrights reserved.

Lesson #13: Involve Your Family in the Ministry/Business Organization.

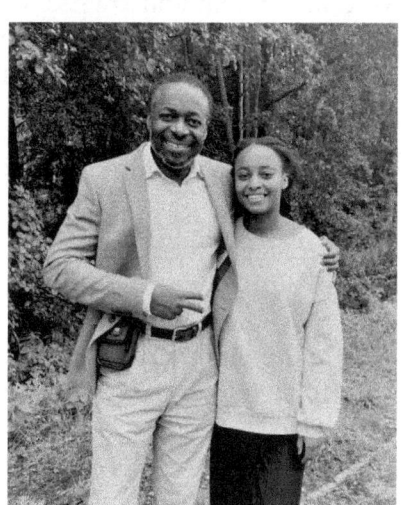

I am writing this page in Lancaster, today – as I arrived the previous day with the rest of the family to celebrate the safe passage of my eldest child from the teenage-years into young adulthood!

Only the unwise *would* bid to do contrary to my learning: Even if you were a sole proprietor, business person or one involved in an itinerant ministry, your immediate family ought to be brought into the knowledge of at least, the fundamental 'basics' of your business/ministerial operations!

It even sounds more logical to me that your spouse necessarily must be involved in the ministry/business you run – to the very extent that God has called and gifted him/her!

God forbid that you are pronounced dead – or become incapacitated in any way; someone from within *your* inner circle ought to be able to operate the enterprise in your absence!

Involving your trusted, beloved, family members in the ministry/business at the initial stage would *not* automatically arrogate them to the helmsman status of the ship's crew! With due diligence and co-operational training, however, they would be able to play a more significant role in the entrenchment of the roots – and the growth of new foliage of the organization's vision!

And while some argue for or against this thought, God has helped me to involve mine, gradually, at each turn of my enterprise. Part of my deliberate "involvement" this weekend was to:

1.) Surprise my big girl with our presence on an unannounced, unexpected visit up north, at her University-town's residence; and,

2.) Grant her once-upon-a-time desire: *"Dad, could you for once leave your grey facial hair and silver tones on your head and beard for all to see?"*

Those weren't far too expensive experiences for either of us: Strong emotional bonds formed with your loved ones will in turn automatically facilitate their bonding with your vision!

FAMILY, MINISTRY, BUSINESS & CORPORATE MATTERS 31

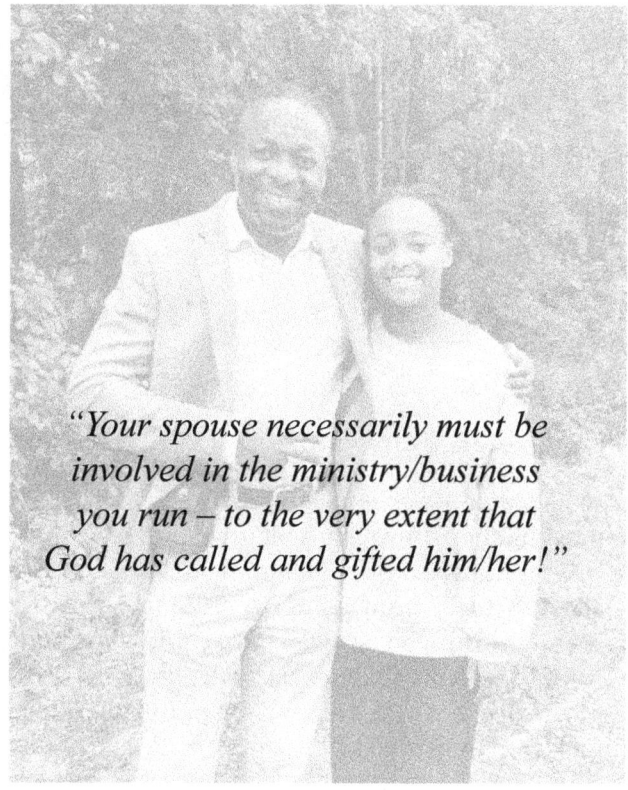

"*Your spouse necessarily must be involved in the ministry/business you run – to the very extent that God has called and gifted him/her!*"

Photo on the preceding page shows Dr. Sammy Joseph and his eldest daughter, Miss Gabriella Joseph; Lancaster, 2018. Copyrights reserved.

Lesson #14: Differentiate Roles in the Family, Ministry/Business.

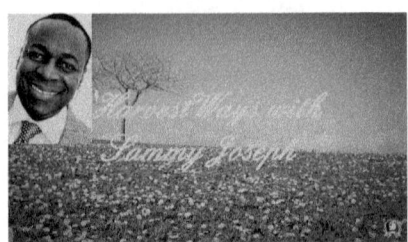

When you play our sermons on the YouTube, this, above, is the most likely picture that will greet and welcome you. Some of you know where our broadcasts are archived at; some do not! Well, I am going to seize the bulls by the horns – and inform you anyway. You could view and subscribe to our YouTube channel *HarvestWays*. Your subscription will ensure that you stay abreast of future uploads or teachings from our ministry!

If you ever heard me preach at our church, at a conference, on the radio – or anywhere else in the world, your spirit would quickly attest to the candid, prophetic messages the Lord has given me to share with the world! Here's just one:

> *"Resist the lure to lump roles together if you would be distinguishable in the family, ministry and business*

circles of influence!"

I just couldn't shout it any louder: *Differentiate roles for your staff – and let each person be very clear as to the specifics of their respective duties!*

I had first tested this rule at home on my five young children as they were raised. And despite children's delinquency, may I add, it *had* worked overall! Delineating boundaries in actual roles and duties had made each child aware of my expectations of them – which by the way had not been low at all! Same rule had worked for me in the ministry. I am certain it will work for you too in your business/organization!

If you still require more information on my viewpoint expressed here, I have written extensively on the issue of separation of the person from his/her title, in my book *GIDEON: Releasing the Potentials Within You*; published by PULSE Publishing House, UK. It is available at *harvestways.org* – and everywhere books are sold online. Order yourself a copy today!

> *"Resist the lure to lump roles together if you would be distinguishable in the family, ministry and business circles of influence!"*

The photo on the preceding page is the familiar, welcoming logo of HarvestWays' YouTube channel that would likely greet you as you click to watch our videos. Copyrighted to Sammy Joseph Ministries.

Lesson #15: Specialize in Your Core; Be it Family, Ministry/Business.

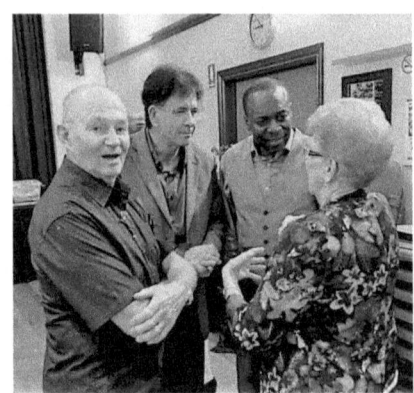

Life is shorter than to be lived doing what you hate doing merely because of the pay. Truth is, if you dared start on what you alone know God had deposited inside of you to do on earth, doors will open, eventually. But you *must* persevere at it – and be full of gusto. Eventually, you will succeed!

To be reckoned a success in the eyes of God – and in this current life, however, you must find that niche you were carved by Heaven to fit into – and fill it with zest!

I love seeing souls arrive into the Kingdom of God.

I love people. I love meeting them and giving – and receiving hugs – and *'Hi five's!'*

I love laughing, heartily. (And if my laughter becomes offensive to you, I would quietly excuse myself from your corner – and continue laughing anyway!)

I love reading – and writing.

I love imparting knowledge and truthfully guiding others in God's wisdom.

I love teaching and prophesying the Word verbally – and non-verbally.

I love the discipline of both a disciplined, studious mind – and life.

I love the presence of God. (But I also love my presence).

I love looking into the camera lenses and posing for a photoshoot. Or better, still, talking! I love to talk. (I talk for a living).

I hate correcting people – even when we all know it's part of a leader's job quotient to be decisive! (But I also love being vulnerable with the right people).

I hate with a passion lies, and liars – and pretenders!

I love my family – and friends.

I love Jesus Christ.

And on and on, I may continue!

What am I trying to pass across to you?

Be passionate about who you are. Don't you dare let death catch you out having *not* executed Heaven's blueprint for your life. That would be tragically fatal!

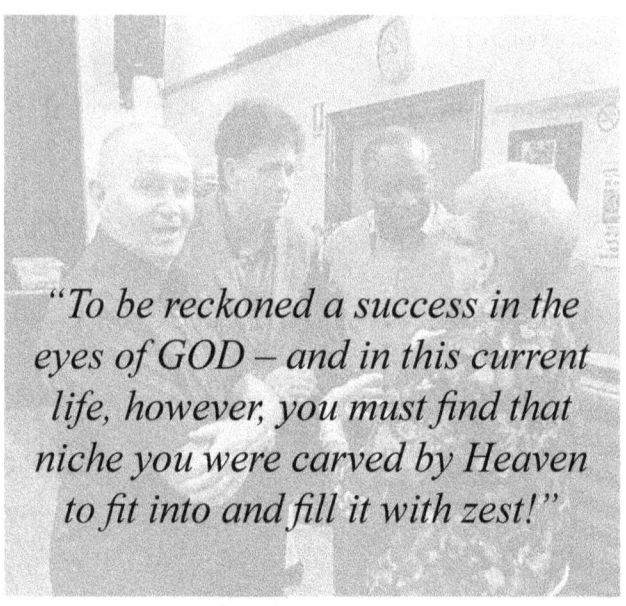

"To be reckoned a success in the eyes of GOD – and in this current life, however, you must find that niche you were carved by Heaven to fit into and fill it with zest!"

The original photograph was taken during the Int'l Experience Harvestways Conference, Tamborine, Queensland, Australia, February 2018. Copyrighted; Sammy Joseph Ministries. (The middle-aged lady and her husband had traveled two hours and booked a local guest house to partake of Dr. Sammy Joseph's services that weekend. She had testified of "a thick lump dissolving from my breast after Dr. Joseph had laid hands upon my head and prayed for me!" Her husband had looked at the camera while the host pastor, Chris Maynard, and Dr. Joseph had looked on in awe of the potency of our Father-God!)

Lesson #16: Don't let a Crushing Cause You an Offense against Christ Jesus.

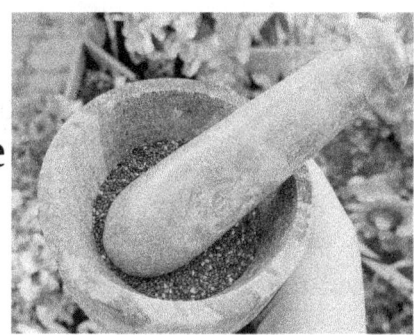

Not all crushing is from the devil! Or did you think otherwise?

A crushing could indeed be a self-inflicted punishment – for your lack of better judgment – for which you must accept the responsibility thereof! When anyone uses his/her mouth to inflict a curse upon himself/herself, he or she has gone against the teaching of the Scripture in *Proverbs 18:21*. Or say for example, when another casts all restraints to the winds – and takes a huge loan against their credit on consumer-goods, that's the beginning of the end of their financial freedom!

Then also, the wicked one – Satan – comes crashing at the holy seed! Here's the truth:

> *"Satan crushes upon every saint in order to prevent*

God's good ore inherent in each, from flowing out!"

But he always makes that mistake – because that which Satan planned for our evil, our God usually always turns around for our good | *Genesis 50:30 & Romans 8:28.*

However, some 'crushings' are from Father-God!

Have you seen those controlled experiment car-crashes carried out by car manufacturing giants just before the new model gets released into the auto market world in countless millions?

In a similar – but even safer – way, our Father-God too carefully fore-plans and executes His test-crashes on us and our unaligned desires! His very goal is to refine the ore in us His saints, before releasing it to the world through us!

Whichever of these 'crushings' you had experienced, currently are experiencing or will experience; can I plead with you to never let a 'crushing' catch you unawares, cause you an offense – or turn your back against the Lord?

Patiently offer unto Him your thanksgiving – even in the doldrums! Your *'westerly'* will surely breeze again.

P.S:

And may I just quickly add that the greater the crushing, the costlier the ore/anointing to be released forth!

"Satan crushes upon every saint in order to prevent God's good ore inherent in each, from flowing out!"

Original photo depicting the crushing of dried seeds; courtesy SJM, Birmingham, England.

Lesson #17:
If God promised it, He will Deliver it! Trust Him through – and thoroughly!

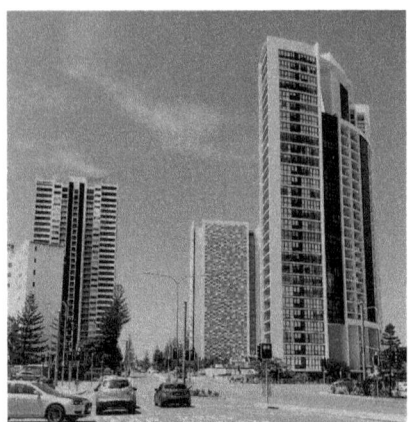

T

This is one of the photos I took in Gold Coast, Queensland, Australia, February 2018. My host had driven me out on this day to sightsee the city. This is the downtown, called *Surfers' Paradise*. It boasts of some of the tallest buildings in the world – inhabited by the world's richest and most affluent. It is this picture that alights on my mind as I write *Lesson #17*. Here it is:

> "If God promised it, He will deliver it! Trust Him through – and thoroughly!"

Let's face the reality: Life will *never* be fair for the majority in the world.

Some of you have taken some ram-battering thus far; and, thus are confused. All that remains is the last breath in your lungs! But with that very last breath, I will ask you to wait on God for the delivery of the promise! Don't lose hope, dear one! Father-God specializes in restoring double-fold to all those who patiently, rejoicingly, await His salvation. These are they Prophet Zechariah envisioned as *"prisoners of hope"* in his book, *Zechariah 9:12*.

God saved me at the tender age of three – and called me *"an evangelist and a prophet unto the nations"* at age five. No one was there! He baptized and filled me with the Holy Spirit with the evidence of speaking in tongues at eleven in the boarding school without anyone laying hands upon me. My first public major sermon was delivered at twenty-five to a packed hall audience of just above three-hundred youths! Thereafter, He opened the doors to major countries of the world for me to speak at. Yet, as I write today, there are aspirations yet to be fulfilled, heights yet to conquer – and soils I am yet to set foot upon!

You see, God's execution of visions to humans are appointed to be fulfilled at designated times and seasons. I run His errands – inclusive of all the variables that could occur – not forgetting the delays caused by the hosts of hell, digressions caused by my human-nature and detours caused by my less-than-fortunate choices! God's grace accommodates every variable!

I had laid somewhat in the doldrums of life for about a decade until November 2014 when God had re-visited His vision unto me. He had said He was ready to take the *Experience HarvestWays Conference* from pole to pole; from the east to the west of the earth, and from the north to the south!

By faith alone – not having celebrated the fourth year of God's re-visitation of this vision in 2018 – I have taken the

Gospel to four of the seven continents of the world, transforming lives and the destinies of peoples, businesses, families, ministries, and churches! (And we really haven't started yet!) That was the reason I penned that you too wait for your *due* season – with the emphasis on the word *"due."*

Do *not* be in a hurry, dear weary soul!

God never forgot His promises. (Never you forget yours.)

Be always ready. He will send for you. He will deliver you. He will deliver *to* you.

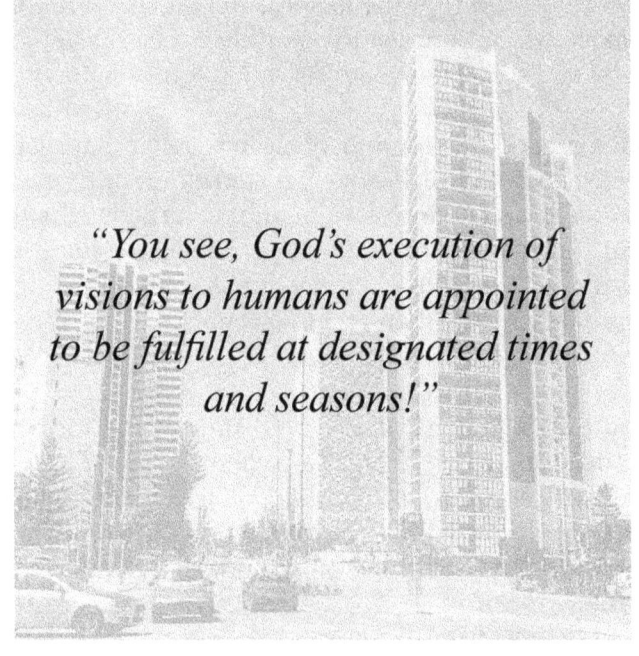

"You see, God's execution of visions to humans are appointed to be fulfilled at designated times and seasons!"

Original photo of Broadbeach/Surfers' Paradise, Gold Coast, Australia. One of these buildings is the world's second tallest building. Copyrights; SJM, England.

Lesson #18: Be Ruthless with Weeds Generally wherever They're found; Either in a Family, Ministry/ Business.

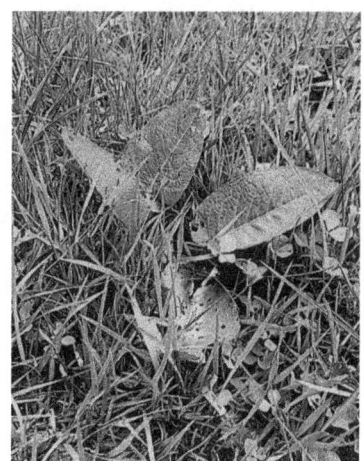

That picture above is that of a dock-leaf weed growing among a lush, green grass in my garden. This one lesson is short! Colloquially, you planted wheat. You expected only wheat to grow. They grew – but weeds showed up too. Unfortunately, every time weeds are ready to spread, they display their colorful flowers – and dispositions! If you're inexperienced at weeding them, a single touch disposes off the ripened seeds, air-borne most times. That touch helps spread farther, their growth!

Dock-leaf weed is one of the most toxic types of weed-plants prone to mass-invasion of your garden in no time *if* let alone! They require the attention of surgical gardeners who would completely take care of them from the roots!

In the same token, it may be tough on your financial disposition in the short run, but sparing *any* weed a deep uprooting should only spell more difficulty and a stretch on both your resources and the well-being of your wheat/crop in the long run!

I have learned with the advent of time that whenever you gain sight – or sense – of a *weed-sprout* near your marriage, home, children, ministry or business; it matters not the depth, the width or the height of your emotional connectivity to that tap-rooted human weed, you know how ruthless you ought to get with its uprooting!

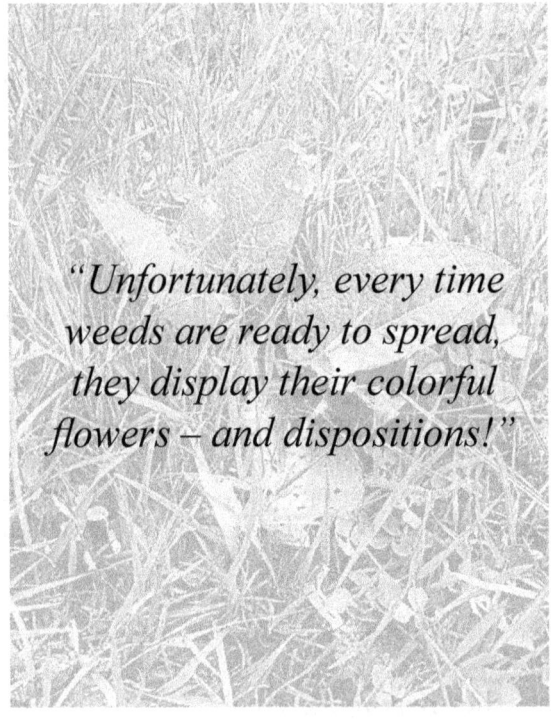

"Unfortunately, every time weeds are ready to spread, they display their colorful flowers – and dispositions!"

The photo on the preceding page is a dock-leaf shoot sprouting amidst luxuriant garden grass courtesy of SJM, Birmingham, England. Copyrighted.

Lesson #19: Handling a Prodigal's Return to the Fold.

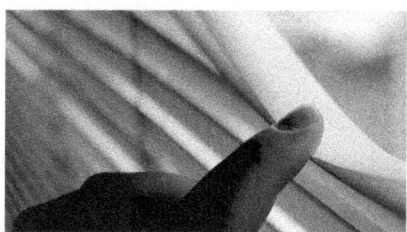

Should the reckless repent, convert and demonstrate genuine, penitent interest in re-joining the mainstream flow of family, friendship, ministry or corporate establishment; they must be jealously guarded against falling into the easy-ready temptations of treachery, ever again! (Notice, I have *not* suggested that they be kept in a confinement, or an isolation of any kind, watched from a closed-circuit television monitor. Or treated suspiciously in any way! Doing so would violate your humaneness towards them as a redeemed, graceful soul.)

What I've advocated is the necessity/need for an entrusted "border agent" to superintend over their activities both spiritually, emotionally and physically. (Refer to *Judges 21:25*).

There must exist – at least – a specified reason why *'retur-*

nees' are so labeled. And that lone reason must not be so easily dismissed or discounted by the head of the family, ministries or business enterprise.

I have learned – as a local pastor with almost three decades of experience – that *returnees* cannot possibly be afforded the liberty of easing in and out of a corporate entity recklessly at will, to the utmost anger of the pure of heart who had – and still have – remained faithful to the house all while long!

True apostles of Christ *"have received grace and the apostleship authority to call for obedience to the faith among all nations, for His name!"* Romans 1:5 | Amplified Version. This is a sound teaching of the Scripture. I do hope you do understand what that verse entails?

> *"Returnees cannot possibly be afforded the liberty of easing in and out of a corporate entity recklessly at will!"*

The original photo on the preceding page depicts a watchful pair of eyes and hands, courtesy SJM, Birmingham, England.

Lesson #20: Understanding Mirages in the Family, Ministry/Business.

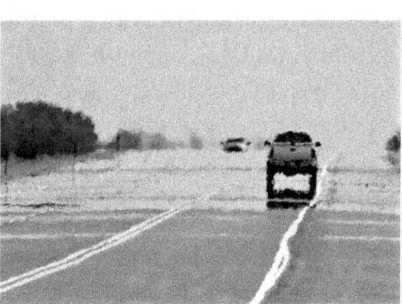

M

Mirages could produce a sight of intrigue, sometimes! They form as a result of air-refraction in the atmosphere!

Let's apply the same principle that forms a mirage on the earth's surface to the truth that exists in the spiritual realm, shall we?

It could become intriguing too, that a person with the call of God upon their life suffered so much pain, neglect, rejection and abandonment at the back of life's desert, that they began to re-think: *'Maybe God hadn't actually called me?'* If adequate spiritual care is not taken, they would soon gradually drift away from the God-given vision; eagerly, in pursuit of mirages!

But wait!

The pursuance of mirages on a calling's journey is the clearest evidence to me, of the devil's throw of a diversionary, tactical, curve-ball at the visionary! If that scheme fails, his next equally diabolical, fiery dart in his weaponry of attacks is a fast, spin-toss of the spirit of frustration – followed either by a jealous, bitterly critical or an unforgiving spirit.

I write about what I *have* partaken of!

But never forget that God always has the scripts of your life firmly, in His hands, dear called-one! Don't be weary. Quench that burning thirst to throw in the towel with the knowledge of God's word: Mirages are *not* oases. They mislead a soul to famish. Avoid distractions like as if they were plagues. Keep journeying, onward. You should arrive at your destination in no time!

> *"The pursuance of mirages on a calling's journey is the clearest evidence to me, of the devil's throw of a diversionary, tactical, curve-ball at a visionary!"*

The mirage picture on the preceding page is copyrighted to Jeffrey Beall, https://geekswipe.net/science/physics/why-do-we-see-mirages accessed, September 26, 2018 at 19.11 hours GMT.

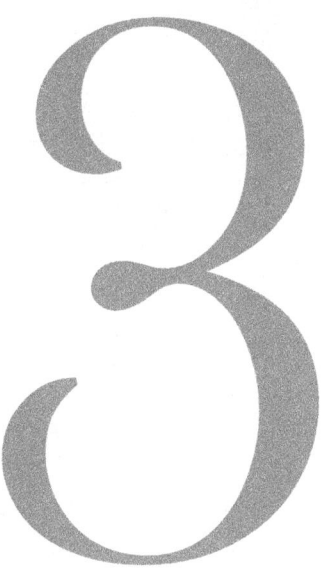

Part Three

Listening for Divine Instructions in Wisdom on Cogent Matters

Lesson #21: Wrathful Fight with God on specific instructions Relating to Family, Ministry/Business.

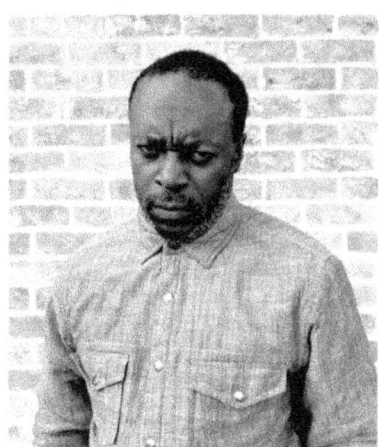

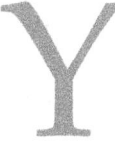

You stripped before a bathroom mirror to have a shower – and took a long, narrow look at the figure standing in front of you. Silver linings are beginning to form on your temples, armpits – and indeed, at other areas!

You look again, this time, retrospectively at your achievements in life. You feel pity for yourself! You felt you're a long way behind others. The unmistakable inner voice of God's Holy Spirit was instructing you otherwise, but you're angry at Him!

Look at that picture again, please; will you? It depicts your angry disposition at God's specific breakthrough-instructions to you regarding either your family, marriage, ministry or business. Your anger may have brooded over His instruction to you to sow a financial seed unto a minister of God – or some ministries! You knew it – but have refused to obey. You have emerged from the quiet room very displeased, angry, and in a fighting disposition. No wonder your heaven hadn't released its rain. For the rebellious will continually inhabit *"a dry land"* | Psalms 68:6.

When will you stop the wrath?

When will you call the truce?

When will you do what God says to you to do – even though it may seem so hard to obey, at the present? There are untold blessings in a life of yielded obedience to Him!

I underwent a very nasty divorce proceeding between 2004 and 2007. I had been physically violated in domestic violence for almost a decade of marriage that had involved suicidal threats from ex-wife, two police arrests and detentions of me without any criminal record ever found or recorded against me. Then, one fall afternoon in 2005 after a most horrific, unprovoked, physical attack on me, I had been convinced:

> *God hates divorce. But He probably hated even much more, the abuse – or the domination – of another and the exposure of innocent children to utter madness!*

I had *had* enough.

I had filed for divorce – and a Restraining Order on her! (That face above could easily have been mine at such an uncommon season of life.)

Thank God for his restorative grace, today. But please, listen to the voice of the Holy Spirit speaking to you through

LISTENING FOR DIVINE INSTRUCTIONS IN WISDOM ON COGENT MATTERS 53

my pen: *"Don't have it your way!"* Acquiesce your will to Divine supremacy! *"Human anger does not achieve God's righteous purpose"* | James 1:20; Good News Translation.

"God hates divorce. But He probably hated even much more, the abuse – or the domination – of another and the exposure of innocent children to utter madness!"

The picture on the preceding page, shows the author modeling an angry face. Copyrights reserved, SJM, Birmingham, England.

Lesson #22: When You've Been Lifted High by God, Never Forget Your Roots!

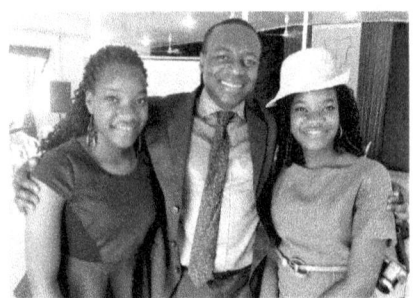

L

Lesson #22 is the second of just two lessons the Lord would have me write on "listening for divine instructions in wisdom on cogent matters." You have read the first. Here's the second:

Aren't you glad you are *not* God?

Probably, if you had been granted the power, you would have wiped out *your* world – many times over because of offense, grudges, and unforgiveness. I am so grateful God did not arrogate to anyone His omnipotence!

I have met and counseled with individuals who in infancy had either been critically abused and possibly forever damaged by the messed-up family set-up's in which they had been raised. The irony is that body-cells, tissues, and bones continue to grow until adulthood, but the spirit in humans may have been stifled at childhood! These were the victims of yester-years who emerged as abusers and predators of today!

But you are *not* created to adopt the victim's mentality. You are a victor because of the faith endowed you by the Son of God, Jesus Christ! A victor's spirit – like Joseph's with the background of a blended, dysfunctional family like Jacob the patriarch's – forgives, and in turn blesses those who had viciously meant him undeterred harm!

Can I ask you by the Holy Spirit: *"Who are those blood-relatives you have damned to hell, whom the Spirit of God is repeatedly asking you to open your heart unto – and help raise or pull up?"*

Psalms 133 was one of the songs the Jews had sung as they had climbed the treacherous bypass heights onto Jerusalem. Those songs had never failed to lift up their spirit as they had journeyed onward in high anticipation. A verse of that short song says wherever siblings dwell together in unity, there, God *"bestows His blessing, even life forevermore."*

I have encountered two or three rich, bitter individuals at their deathbeds. No one had come to see them. They had died miserable, lonely deaths.

Don't cut your reasonable family members off. If you do, you too are likely going to experience a miserable, lonely, forsaken end!

Listen to the voice of God: Cease warfare – and the retaliation against those who had mistreated and abused you. Let the love of God cause you to forgive, forget – and *"cover a multitude of sins"* | 1 Peter 4:8. If you are so mean-spirited, hand them over to God in prayers for a justifiable retribution!

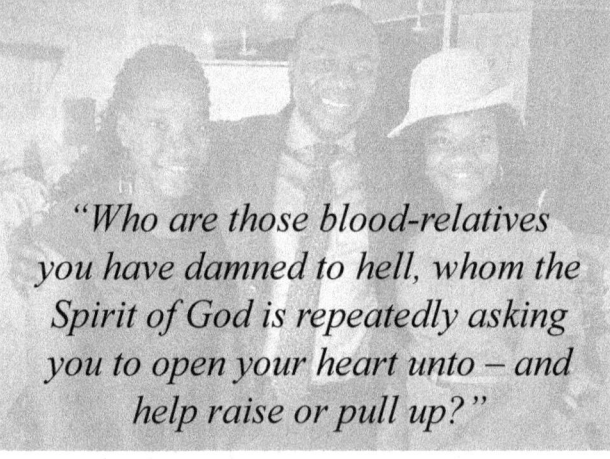

"Who are those blood-relatives you have damned to hell, whom the Spirit of God is repeatedly asking you to open your heart unto – and help raise or pull up?"

In the original picture on the preceding page, Dr. Sammy Joseph poses with his twin-nieces; Ife, Nigeria, November 2017. Copyrights reserved.

■ Part Four

Friends Contrasted with Fiends

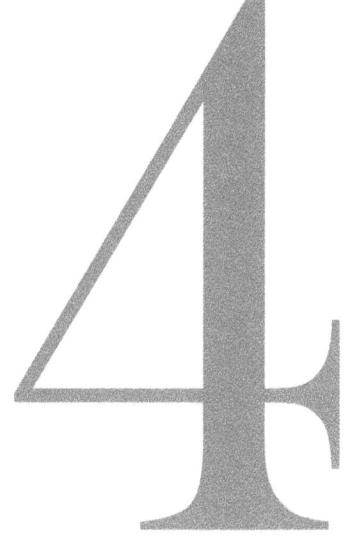

Lesson #23: Contrasting of the word "Friend" with "Fiend."

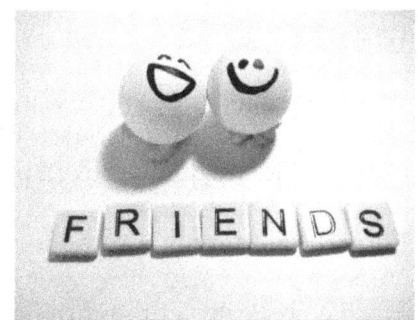

Having been un-burdened by the urgent, cogent instructions of the Lord, I shall on the next few pages be sharing just a few of the many great lessons I've learned about 'true friendship' contrasted with 'untrue friendship'. I shall engage the letters in the word 'friends', as an acronym: *"F.R.I.E.N.D.S"*

Are you ready for *Lesson 23* – the very first lesson in friendship?

Then, look at those two friends up there in the picture: One is a happy face. The other, a frowning face. They obviously do *not* look well-suited for each other! The biblical term for this kind of relationship is *"unequal yoke"* | See *2 Corinthians 6:14.*

Unbelievably, sadly enough, the *happy, sunshine* fella

would constitute an unbeknown hinderance to the *heavy, overcast* fellow. Their friendship would undoubtedly soon turn fiendish!

If you were like me, you'd want to be really, very careful choosing friends. You wouldn't be choosing un-balanced, out-of-joint, unequally-yoked personalities as friends!

Enough said for now! I'd be back on the next page!

Have a great day – or night!

"If you were like me, you'd want to be really, very careful choosing friends."

Photo on the preceding page shows two faces proposing friendship!

Lesson #24: "F" stands for "Fierce Loyalty."

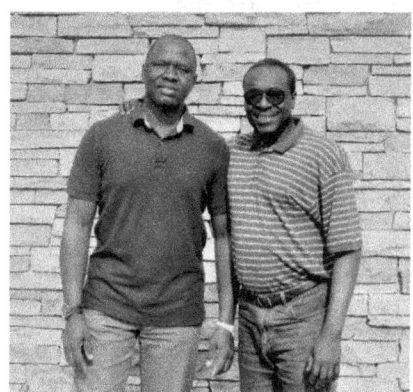

I have a friend I have been in an ever-rewarding friendship with, for over thirty-five years. He defined the meaning of "friendship" to me in those early teenage years. He had looked at me in the eye and said: *"A true friend is always fiercely loyal!"* We had met at barely fifteen years old, I being a few months older!

Ollie was from a Moslem upbringing and had been strong in his faith. Whenever we had dabbled into the discussion about our different faiths, he had always said I would convert to his. I had prophesied to him God's hands were upon him as he had been separated as a chosen vessel unto Him from the womb. *"You will someday become a pastor,"* I'd always ended our conversations bordering on the faith with.

We grew in loyalty and friendship with each other over

the years. Ours was a tested and proven brotherly love; admiration, and respect.

Towards the end of our University academic years, however, I had sat down with him – and for the last time explained the urgency of his need to accept Christ Jesus into his heart. When he had refused, I had blatantly told him: *"Your refusal to accept the Lord Jesus is an automatic sentence to the condemnation of hellfire as the Holy Bible teaches in John 3:16-20. Ollie, I am sorry, but I cannot furthermore pledge allegiance to you other than a commitment to ongoing further prayers."*

He had replied to me: *"Sammy, you are the particular one going to Satan's hell; you watch!"* And at that, I had decided to call it quits.

We had quit friendship until about five or six years later when Ollie had re-visited my house on an impromptu visit. As I'd gazed at him thirty meters away from my door, I had shouted out the first question. Your guess of that question should be correct: I had asked: *"Am I still the one going to hell, Ollie?"*

With wet eyes and a head shaken in the non-affirmative, he had replied: *"Neither of us is going to hell, Sammy; I am now a born-again child of God!"* That had sounded like music to my ears. We had hugged – and had automatically picked up from where we'd cooled off in the previous years.

Today, Ollie, his wife, and four children live in Canada – having adopted Canada as their home. He is the pastoral counseling head of his church. My joy as that child-prophet still knows no bounds! Our friendship too knows no limit!

In retrospect, let me re-define what the word "friend" means to me: *"A friend is one whom I give the advantage unto freely, because my heart fiercely gives it!"*

True friendship will cost you. It will demand of you, commitment and fierce loyalty. It will break, mend and heal your tiny heart, expanding it to love ever more so fiercely. The fierceness of loyalty will compel you to lay down 'stuff' you never thought you had. It will bless you tremendously beyond measure, in the long run!

As God began opening doors unto our ministries across the world, He is expanding ever so widely both the span and the scope of my friendships. Furthermore, He is enlarging my capacity to nurture more genuine friendships. He may be bringing *you* and *I* in contact soon enough!

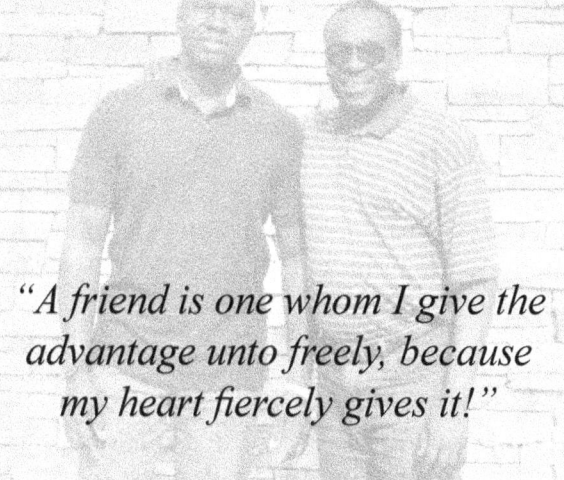

"A friend is one whom I give the advantage unto freely, because my heart fiercely gives it!"

In the original photo, Dr. Sammy Joseph poses with his teenagerhood friend, Ollie, on a visit to Niagara Falls, Ontario, Canada, June 2013. Copyrighted.

Lesson #25: "R" stands for "Ruthlessness in Attracting – and Keeping Friends!"

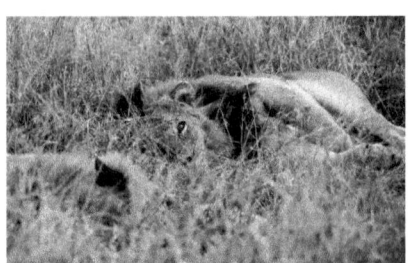

Your disposition may be diametrically varied to mine, but that's fine. The Bible says: *"As water reflects the face, so does a man's heart, to him"* | Proverbs 27:19. In other words, you see in another what you see in you!

Can I further simplify?

A person's spirit can only attract, in true friendship, who they truly are | 1 Corinthians 2:11. Once or twice though, a crooked, half-baked individual like Ephraim may want to draw upon your attention for friendship. It seems certain to me that a friendship pact with an Ephraim-individual should *never* be signed! Because that friendship if entered into through naivety, will soon turn *fiendish*. I learned that once God reveals to you, your pathways are uneven, you carefully, ruthlessly take off!

I once had a lying cheat closing in upon my inner circle of friends, a decade ago. His moves were sleek and full of subtlety. Since I was not a cheat, nor ever a criminal, my spirit produced the ultimate maneuver of ruthlessness on his person. He was toppled while he sat unexpecting *the* least trouble. I had wiped him off my mind as the cool, morning water dissolves – and washes dirt and oil off a visage!

A total cleansing is what the eyes need for the sharpest vision. Eyes give light to the entire body. If therefore your vision is uninhibited, see how much light will flood your life | *Matthew 6:22*. You probably cannot mix a hue of black paint with silk diamond white – and emerge with full, diamond, silk-white color upon your wall! Take cue! Don't you ever let no "so-called" friend fool you. I never granted that *fiend* an audience again, until this very day! My very few friends and I hold each other to strictly high levels of Godly expectations. We also extend grace unto one another in our crucial times of need! A slight, evil communication will taint your good manners *if* you let it!

> *"I learned that once God reveals to you, your pathways are uneven, you carefully, ruthlessly take off before deeper commitments are made!"*

Photo: A picture of two lionesses in the wild who had ruthlessly fended off an intruding lion to protect their cubs.

Lesson #26: "I" stands for "Intricate Interest."

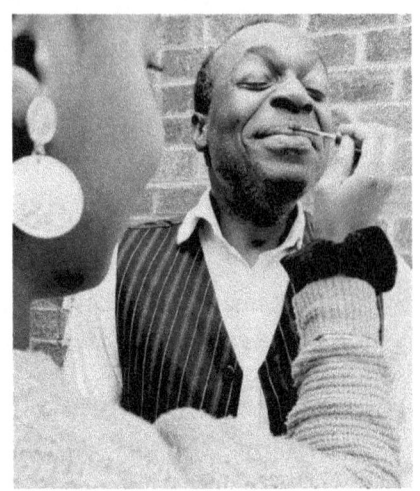

I

It's *not* rocket science, you know! If you're genuinely intending to become friends with someone, you would develop an intricate interest in getting to know them. You will note their 'likes' and 'dislikes', to say the very least! You will endeavor to know their tastes. You will possess a working knowledge of their personality! You will know what irritates – or excites them!

My closest friends know me – and I, them! In addition, they know that I love to play 'monkey-ish' pranks. So, they play it on me too! My children especially – when growing up – had outplayed me on my invention! They still sometimes do. They would say something like this: *"Dad, it's your turn. So, close your eyes too ..."* And I've had to obey their wishes!

That picture above was taken by my second daughter,

Prissy. It was impromptu – and totally unrehearsed. At least, from my end. Well, maybe the two sisters had exchanged notes on what pranks they were about to play on me. Anyway, I had fallen captive to their pranks, unknowingly!

Some of you parents have stiffened up on enjoying life with your kids. And you really need to loosen up. You've chosen rather to remain forever authoritative in those rapidly growing and changing young lives: You've totally missed the point. That's why you lose those children in the mid-adult phase of development!

If you've done a fairly thorough, sincere, honest and faithful parenting; by eighteen years of age, your relationship with each of your children ought to be transitioning into an ever-closer, intimate friendship!

Anyway, back to my story; that day I'd been asked to comply with the pretty ladies' wishes. My senses had been flooded with a sudden premonition. Cajoling emotions had washed over me when the unexpected, cold, first stroke of the brown *Matte* lipstick had hit my lips – and I had taken a lick of a taste!

What am I saying?

I learned that the exchange of money and gift expressions of love in friendship are great – and essential. But greater still is a friend's faithful observance of the other's intricate details, if their friendship would outlast a hundred thousand miles! The Bible says each of us *"is fearfully and intricately created by God"* | Psalms 139:14.

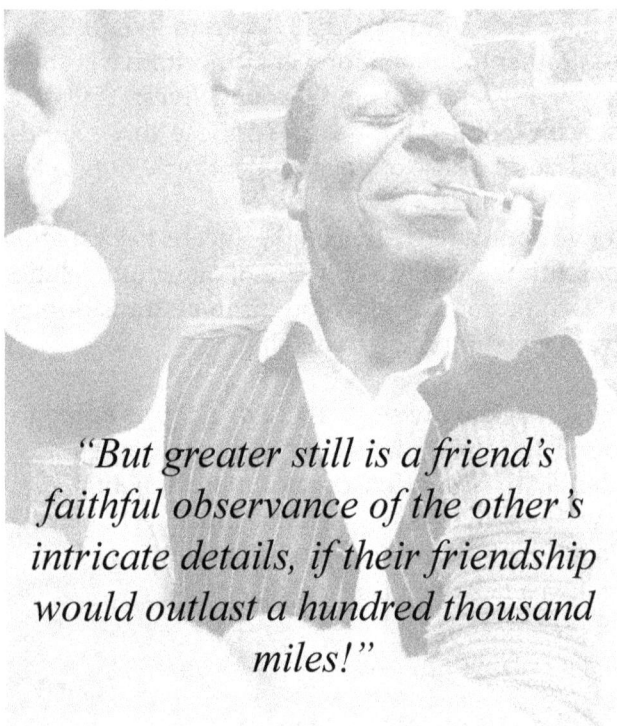

"But greater still is a friend's faithful observance of the other's intricate details, if their friendship would outlast a hundred thousand miles!"

In the original photo on the preceding page, Gabby plays a prank on Dad. Copyrights, SJM, Birmingham, England.

Lesson #27: "E" stands for "Expectation of a high Yield of Returns!"

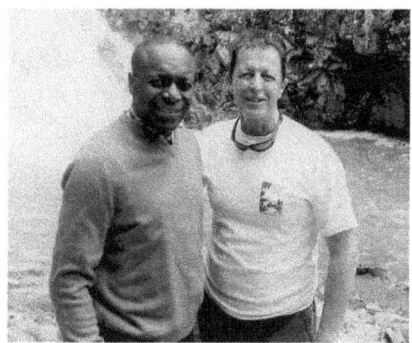

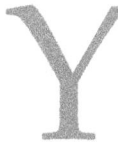

You will recognize the quality of what alliance you're about to enter into by the revealed expectation returns on your investment in that partnership, friendship or alliance! I learned this rule of the thumb in my mid-thirties:

> *"A great friendship will offer you a high yield of returns on your investments while a doomed-to-be-sour friendship will aim at using you solely for its selfish gains!*
>
> *A great friendship will always give the advantage to the other. Not take the advantage."*

A bountiful yield of returns in Godly relationships are like a pair of ear-plugs carrying sweet, soothing, musical melody to the cochlea! Great, rewarding friendships sooth the spirit, melodiously!

Horrible, injurious, malicious fiends too have a tune akin to them. That tune is deception. Power-control. Cohesion. Manipulation. Threatening, and narcissistic manifestations. The ears of your spirit must be attuned to decipher exactly who it is that is plucking your stringed instrument: Is it a "friend" – or a "fiend"?

The disciples led by impetuous Peter had held Jesus to a high yield of returns at His beckon to them to follow Him. Peter had asked: *"What's in this for us that have left all behind, for Your sake?"* | *Matthew 19:27*. The Master Jesus had assured him: *"You who leave all to follow Me; I assure you a hundred-fold return – and folds of hundreds on your investments, both in this present life and in that which is to come!"*

But here's another twist to your returns on investment: Some capricious individuals posing as friends will surely change their words and the terms of the agreement as time goes on. Or they would reiterate the same words of assurance as at the beginning of your 'walk' but never follow through with resultant corresponding actions – even in marriages, ministries and business partnerships! If you'd be wise of heart, you must always remember, God has *not* called you to wrath! Seek therefore peace – and ensue it!

Alternatively, you should be reminded too that you possess the power of the attorney to arrest, handcuff and haul them – and their lies – into the hands of the One Righteous Judge! That ought to be music to their ears!

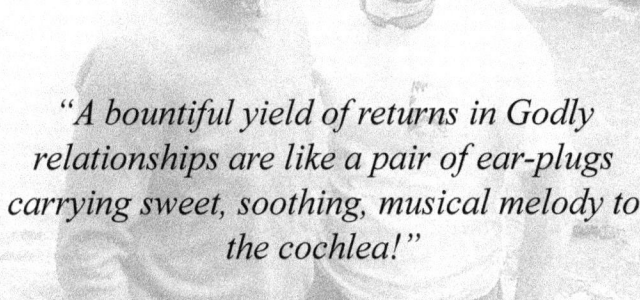

"A bountiful yield of returns in Godly relationships are like a pair of ear-plugs carrying sweet, soothing, musical melody to the cochlea!"

Picture on the preceding page: Dr. Joseph and his appointed tour-guide stopped to pose for a photograph at the Cedar Creek Falls, Mount Tamborine, Queensland, Australia, 2018. Copyrighted. SJM, Birmingham, England.

Lesson #28: "N" stands for "Never become Nebulous in a Friendship."

T

To be *'nebulous'* means to be *'cloudy', 'hazy', 'fuzzy', 'dim', 'shy', 'vague', 'hiding-something back', 'withholding', 'pretentious', 'constrained', 'opaque', 'ambiguous', 'falsely leading another on', etcetera!* You should have overcome any of those abusive traits, a very long time ago – possibly in your mid-teen years of self-discovery!

Can I just 'pick on' *shyness*, to focus upon, for instance?

To be shy is enshrouded in the mystery of being that self-focused, self-centered, self-preserving, self-evolving, confused, proud, adolescent! Apostle Paul says he outgrew youthful, adolescent behaviors to become whom he had eventually become in Christ Jesus!

Being vulnerable does not translate into weakness! Vulnerability is ever going to be one of the greatest strengths and assets you'd be glad you possessed – and had wisely dispossessed yourself off, to the right person, people, ministry or establishment at the right time.

That is a truth I discovered as I journeyed on in life!

If you're rejected after being totally honest, truthful and vulnerable with them, they would become fiendish *if* you pursued that friendship any further. Some other times, rejection will result as a by-product of their lack of your kind of energy, radiance, and stamina! You're loaded with – and worth – far more value than you should avail yourself to any to be dis-respected, used, mis-used, or abused!

Never lose your identity and uniqueness. Never polarize with anyone. Never become nebulous. Be an open, down-to-earth, confident friend.

Say what you may, but I want to daily be a more honest, holier, purer, straighter-to-the-point, no-truth-dresser friend! I made my mind up to be exactly that at fourteen – in 1982.

> *"Say what you may, but I want to daily be a more honest, holier, purer, straighter-to-the-point, no-truth-dresser friend!"*

Original picture of a clear sky and a bright moon over the southern tip of Greenland, June 2013. Copyrights. SJM, Birmingham, England.

Lesson #29:
"D" stands for "Dependability in Friendship."

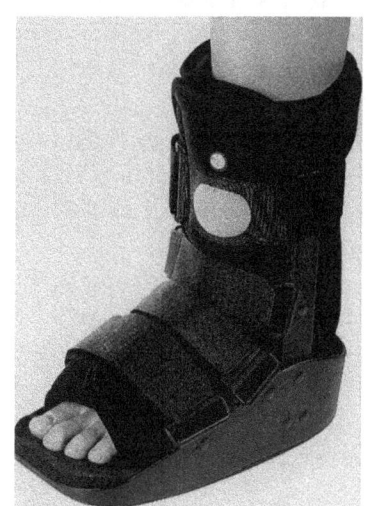

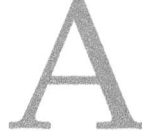

A broken foot. A torn ligament. A pulled muscle. A toothache. Or a jaw pain. Each of these is associated with unbearable pain. (Even a broken zip – or a missing shirt button offers you unreserved embarrassment or shame at the most unexpected times!) Whatever it is, Scripture says: *"Confidence in an unfaithful man in time of trouble is like a broken tooth, and a foot out of joint"* | *Proverbs 25:19*.

To be dependable is to be all that Bill Withers' classic *'Lean On Me'* says. One great attribute a Godly friendship offers is dependability. Others of the same magnitude include: Reliability, compassion, long-suffering – and being solidly there, particularly in the time of trouble!

Fair-weather friends only have sunny dispositions. They do *not* know – neither do want to know – the sublime power that converts silver linings to hues of grey on a life's canvass. These are *not* your friends. They are better suited to be called acquaintances. Trust me, these will *not* be there in your day, week or season of trouble!

When people say they want to be my friend, I smile and ask them like Jesus asked the Zebedee twins: *"Will you also be able to drink the cup assigned me by Heaven?"*

An acquaintance rode in my car in that historic, frigid winter of January 2006. As we slid and plowed along a frozen, icy, uphill road in the city, all of a sudden, my car lost power. That man apologized, excused himself, opened the door and exited. He called a taxi. I never felt like a fool ever before!

Pay attention to in-between-the-lines-speeches, non-verbal looks, body communication, and frivolities!

Are you a broken-tooth friend, an ankle-out-of-joint friend, or a dependable friend? The day, week or season of trouble will reveal!

"One great attribute a Godly friendship offers is dependability."

The photo on the preceding page is of a broken foot in a support, walking boot wear; courtesy SJM, Birmingham, England.

Lesson #30: "S" stands for "Sensitivity in Friendship."

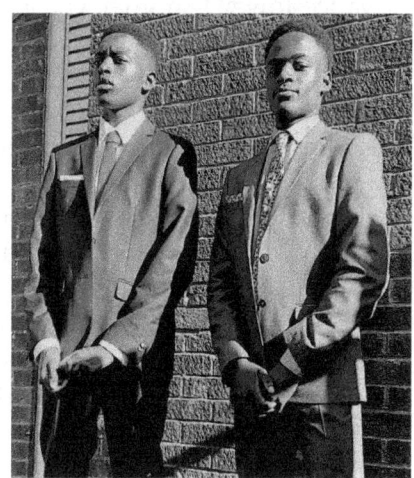

S

Some people are plain touchy. Just over-bearing, over-reacting and senselessly irritable. Such a person won't stand the slightest chance of becoming my friend! Because they are too sensitively serious about themselves that they can't even take a playful touch, a tug at, or a friendly prank. (Maybe they can't even bear the effort at a poke of a joke at themselves?) But I am full of whimsical, harmless fun. That's my emotional make-up. Reasonably and rightly so, they will be quick to say, defensiveness is their emotional composition, too. And that quickly delineates us!

However, a balanced, measured sensitivity is both a perfect defense – and a charming attribute! But you must intuitively know who can and cannot "take" your whims! That ability in itself – to be able to see, sense and gauge when to – or not – be so 'sensitive' about life is the appropriate sensitivity in friendship, I espouse.

You must be sensitive in the spirit too, to know when to advance towards a goal, cause – or altogether withdraw from a pursuit!

Friendship goes through all the seasons. You must be sensitive enough to acknowledge that universal truth!

You must be sensible enough to *not* break trust in friendships. If you did, you must be held self-accountable that you probably couldn't continue to be friends with those you betrayed with a rascally behavior!

You must be courteous enough to know *when* to hold the muscle in your mouth *if* a friend suffers a bereavement, loss – or calamity. Never affirm to them: *"I warned you so!"*

Be sensitive.

Be intuitive.

Be a friend that cares.

Remember, you don't always have to have the last word!

Enough word is said to the wise!

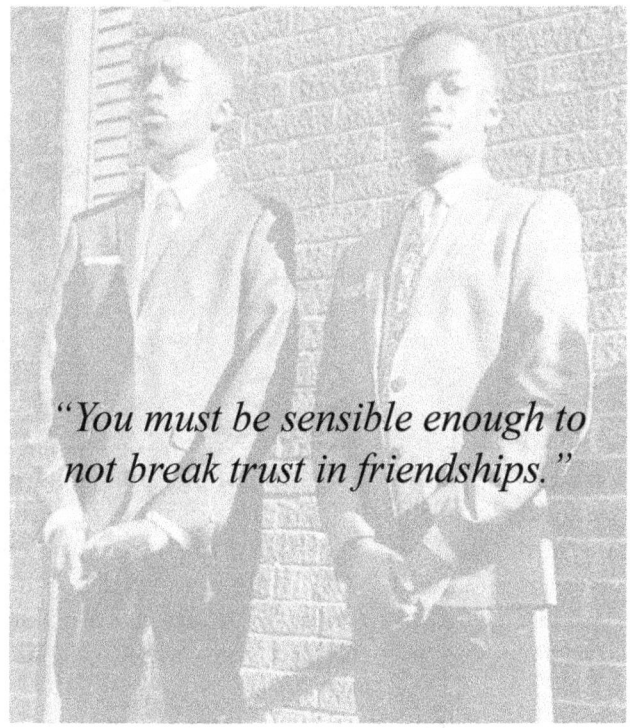

*Original photo: Twin-brothers, David and Daniel model sensitivity in friendship.
Copyright. Gabby Studios, Lancaster, England.*

Lesson #31: Boundaries & Confrontations in Friendship.

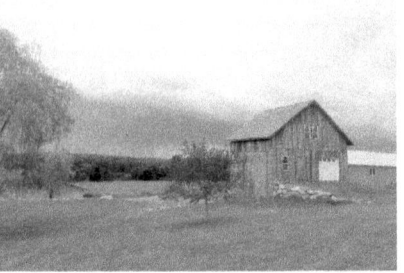

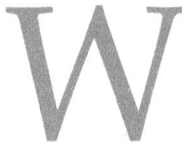

Without having a necessity to dabble into the political quagmire regarding erecting or not erecting national boundaries, may I just quip that every sovereign entity from time immemorial had always observed boundary-markers. Boundary or territory-markers are in place to prevent an aggression – and/or a transgression.

Transgression is the sin of *"going beyond one's bounds."* Most of you growing up in sensitive areas having visited offices in those precincts must have seen the sign hugely displayed: *"Out of Bounds to Non-Staff."*

Boundaries mark borders. You may safely cross them only *if* you are expressly permitted by the owner's authority to do so! Same as in true friendships.

In a true friendship, a boundary demarcates the extent of tolerance that a friend would permit you to explore! Yet, 'boundary' is a word almost everyone is afraid of! But why?

Many are afraid of boundaries because they are ill-disciplined to stay within the perimeter of their bounds! Some are afraid of being caught crossing their friend's boundaries as illegal aliens! Many more have retained sketches of the shame and embarrassment that had ensued following their parents' prosecution and punishment, trafficking away another's boundaries as they grew up! Above all, most people prefer there be no boundaries at all so that there would be no legitimacy of prosecution of a transgression offense. Lack of boundaries surely leads to the commencement of the abuse of legal permit, license or authorization!

A true friendship, however, is comparable to iron sharpening iron: *"As iron sharpens iron, so a man sharpens the countenance of his friend"* | Proverbs 27:17. Instead of drowning in guilt and shame, a true friend succors – and helps you respect their boundaries! (And vice versa!)

Almost everyone hates confrontation. And that includes me. But in my half-a-century experience on earth, I have come to realize that confrontations are a necessary, intrinsic part of healthy friendships/relationships if approached rightly!

Successful parenting, ministries, and marriages cannot be achieved by ducking behavioral issues and pretending as to just wish them away. No; boundaries check the illegal flow of "alien" thoughts and deeds in any healthy venture. Humble confrontations in love act as a mammography screening for the protection of the life of that friendship!

Do you agree?

Write me a feedback. My addresses are at the back of the book.

"Boundaries mark borders. You may only cross them only if they are opened unto you to safely cross."

The photograph on the preceding page reveals a beautiful, isolated, fenceless dwelling house in Iowa, the USA. Copyright permission given by Barbara McCrary.

Lesson #32: 'Kitty-Katty' Friends!

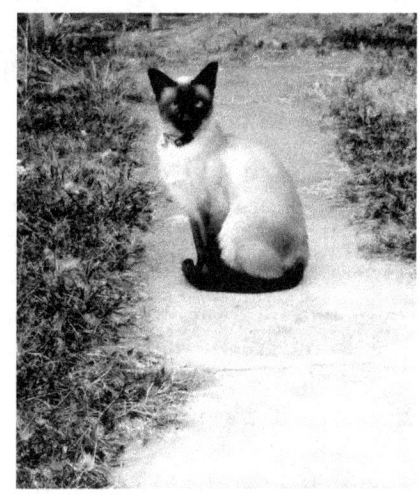

You and I have experienced the unexpected calls from telemarketing companies sounding friendly. We have been irritated, afterward! They've earned the name we call them: Cold-callers! And why not call a cold, "kitty-Katty" friend what he/she is?

You see that dude out there sitting so anxiously in my garden? He is James; my neighbor's, handsome, Jack Point Siamese cat. He's got deep blue eyes and a lovely, sleek, svelte body. His looks, however, betray his rascal behavior!

James loves to stealth into my kitchen – and help himself out of the pot, with chicken-breast chunks from my ration anytime my back door had been left open, particularly in the rising temperatures of the spring and summer months. He's anointed to be both agile and swift. He is equipped with grace to jump out the window if happened upon, find a sitting position from where he licks his lips, acting as if nothing drastic had ever happened! I call him my *kitty-Katty* friend!

Look more carefully, you too would see anointed, human-version, *kitty-Katty* friends in your circle of friends. If you thought I was lying, just look carefully again: *kitty-Katty* friends love to snatch up at advantages and opportunities! They will take-off at your approaching footstalls, acting as if nothing drastic had happened! Well, if you were like me, you'd ensure that that was the very last advantage they ever seized upon!

Here's the Godly deal: When offered an advantage by a friend, be grateful! Receive it graciously but also outsource another way to complement their offer. That's the spirit of true friendship!

When you're also receiving your friend's offer of help, please ensure that you are very considerate in the taking! Do not be greedy at the offer. Be magnanimous. It may just be the iceberg-tip advantage you've greedily snapped upon like a hungry Grouper fish in the swamps when indeed, Father-God had originally intended for you, a mammoth catch in the open ocean!

Don't eat your tomorrow with your today! Desist from growing your appetite into that of a fat, *kitty-Katty* friend!

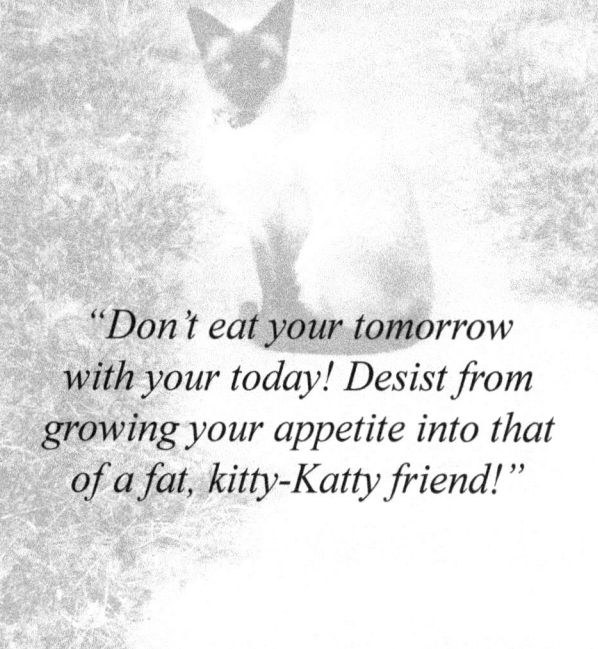

The original photograph overleaf unveils Dr. Sammy Joseph's neighbor's cat, James; in Birmingham, England. Copyrighted, SJM.

PART FIVE

Single, Engaged, Married, Sex and Sexuality

Lesson #33: Complete Singleness.

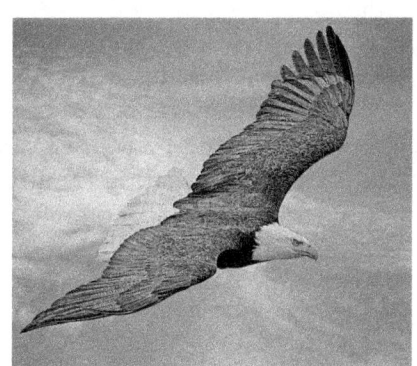

There weren't many knowledgeable teachers of the Word in those days in the eighties when I was growing up into a young man. We only had spiritually-minded teachers who were few, far apart – and unreachable!

I was naive and inexperienced in matters concerning the emotional make-up of humans. In fact, I was just understanding my own emotional make-up, too. By the mid-eighties when I began studying for my first degree at the University, I had not met a member of the opposite sex who had not liked me! (Unfortunately, though, I had not one single, exclusive female called "a girlfriend" as is referred to, today!) I had been consumed primarily with studies. In my spare time however, I had played hockey, sang in an award-winning choir, and prepared for the ministry writing or attending outreaches! The females who had had their eyes *on* me had almost crucified me for an almost, non-existent, social life!

In retrospect, I think that was a blessing in disguise, for that was the season of life wherein my personality had been cast. Those were the days entire chapters of the *Synoptic Gospels* and some books of Psalms had been memorized – and recalled verbatim. I found out these portions, never left me, even up until today! Deferred, delayed gratification in the "normal and ordinary" had had to pave way for the super-normal and the extra-ordinary High calling! It was my best season of *self-discovery* and *self-knowledge*!

Today, I have encountered some unmarried individuals, who at past forty, still haven't a clue about their self-knowledge, let alone, the discovery of their inner yearning! But they are either aggressively finding love – or passively awaiting love to find them!

I fault neither!

What I fault is a person with multiple personalities; one with a confused identity, un-intelligible about, and incomplete in themselves, claiming singleness and expecting true love to find them! Such had better be advised of Apostle Paul who had gone into the seclusion of the Arabian Desert for three years, just to spend time with both himself – and His Lord after his calling, in his bid to self-discover!

I boldly submit to you: No one could be said to be "single" who had not first been complete on their own!

"I boldly submit to you, no one could be said to be "single" who had not first been complete on their own!"

Original photograph: A young Bald Eagle on a self-discovery flight over Paris, Ontario, Canada.
Credit: Gigi Rossignol, for SJM, Copyrighted.

Lesson #34:
Be intently Focused on Hearing from God by Yourself.

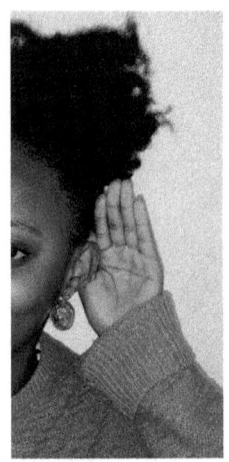

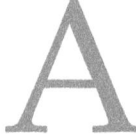

An intrinsic part of integral wholeness is an individual's ability to distinctly hear from God! If you have not figured out how to clearly listen to the voice of the Spirit, your destiny as a Christian is opened to manipulations by the devil, his agents – and spiritist-charlatans!

Wholeness attracts wholeness. Nasty attracts nasty. You may not entirely agree with me, but a person can only attract the kind of spirit they are. Because you see, in the spirit realm, all things are glaringly open, transparent, and un-hidden. If you're pure and prayerful, the very likelihood is that your spirit will attract the same as you. If you discover you attracted otherwise, it is either because the enemy of your soul is insidiously setting you up for a massive destiny-detour, or you are negligent in prayers!

When eventually you've decided who to allow into your life – and that's a decision you should exclusively take unto the Lord in prayers; *you* alone will be responsible for that decision. I appreciate the concerns of biological mothers and siblings in particular, in advising you about your final choice of a spouse after dating. But again, I feel so strongly that if you post the bonds of your future into the hands of familial and siblings' judgments, that's what you will live with for the rest of your life.

Spiritual parents surely can guide in your decision making. That ought to be the exact length of the reins and the bridle they should be entitled to: Pray, guide in intercessory prayers and offer you sound counsel! I have seen spiritual parents who had un-intentionally misguided their flock because they didn't want to be bereft of them since the female usually leaves their ministries/church to join her spouse's. That is spiritual robbery!

If you would be focused; intently focused upon the Lord alone, He will guide you. And *you* alone, will have to follow that guidance.

While it's good that a proposed suitor has going for him a job/viable job-prospect, please do *not* base all your assumptions of their potentials upon what they currently possess or do *not* possess; who they currently are or are *not* in societal status rankings. Intently seek Father-God's face alone – and be fully persuaded in the spirit of your mind, to do whatever He alone asks of you! Banish out of reach human-spirit talks. Never succumb to a familiar spirit's voice!

Be intently focused on listening alone, to the Divine voice speaking from the inside of you *if* you're a child of God | *Romans 14:5.*

"If you have not figured out how to clearly listen to the voice of the Spirit, your destiny as a Christian is opened to manipulations by the devil, his agents – and spiritist-charlatans!"

Original photo: A young lady's hand is cupped behind the ear for clarity of hearing; courtesy SJM, Birmingham, England.

Lesson #35: When She is Genuinely interested in You!

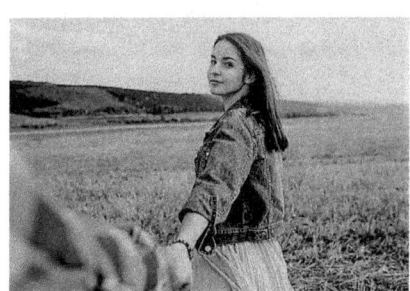

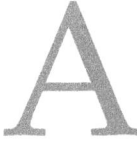

A member of my readership audience asks: *"What signs does a lady give me in order to let me be aware that she's romantically interested in me?"* Therefore, I will devote this lesson to addressing his question!

First and foremost, I'd love you to note that the female species is a gender of special intrigue. No male may totally be able to convincingly say he knows how to perfectly decode the romantic signs a lady who is interested in him gives off! Love-interest signs vary from lady to lady. But here are some telling signs:

1.) She will let you know she's single – and available to be pursued by you: Depending upon her cultural background, she may not aggressively pursue you. In fact, she could tactically, deliberately, withdraw away from showing you deep affectionate interest so that you, the male, may do the pursuing! (I hope you don't miss her vital signs!)

2.) This pretty lady will directly – or indirectly inform you that she has you on her mind.

3.) She will test your affection.

4.) She will not play mind games with your heart: That means she will not 'toy with your head, mind, and emotions.'

5.) If you pass her test, she will begin to open up her life to you, gradually. She will not barrage you with TMI – too much information – all at once. She will open up to you, systematically.

6.) She will honor, respect and treat you like a king.

7.) She will never be too busy to make time out to be with you – no matter how busy she is.

8.) She will be eager to introduce you to her family members and friends.

9.) She is a Godly, God-fearing lady; she will not seduce you in any way: Not even through provocative dressing, pornography – or the offers of her body for your use!

10.) Lastly, she will so gloriously intercede for you before the Lord!

"She will test your affection."

Photo: A young lover-lady leads her date into an open field.

Lesson #36: When He is Genuinely interested in You!

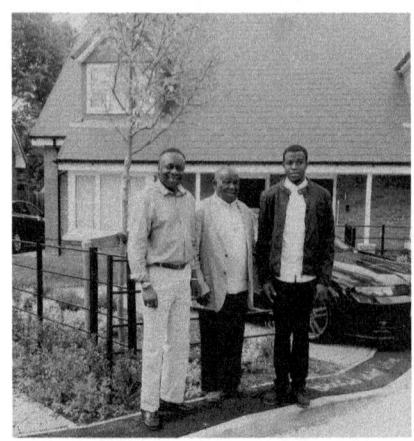

Since the sexes are complementary one to the other, these are some of the signs a female would receive from a genuine male who is romantically interested in her:

1.) He will be *passionately devoted* to you, letting you know that he is into you if the Lord has revealed you to him, as the potential one to pursue. A real man does *not* have a problem in showing and declaring openly to the female he has interest in, his love. Only players will do otherwise.

2.) He will take *the slightest hint from his preferred female to "Come on" as a challenge for a hot pursuit*. He may eventually smother her with love. He will have you on his mind too; not in an obsessive way, but in that special way that he would want to ensure that the hunt is on, with a never-ending appeal in sight!

3.) He will *rise to the female's test of his affection*. If he's like me, he'd bore you with detailed answers to every question. (This could be a misconstrued strength by most females because it's exactly the way 'fakes' behave. In other words, don't sound like too good to be true when you are indeed way, farther much more, than could be disbelieved!)

4.) This is a man of God. *He will not play mind games; neither will he 'play' with the lady's head, mind, and/or emotions.*

5.) If he's ready for marriage, you won't be the one to ask him to take you to the altar. *He will propose marriage to you in no time – and ask to meet your parent(s).* And if he's busy studying, he would ask if you could wait for him to graduate and settle into a job, before proposing marriage to you.

6.) *He will honor, protect, serve and treat you like a queen.* He will not entrap or suffocate you with gifts. Irrespective of his culture – which he will gratefully explain to you – he will buy you gifts and expect you to appreciate the gifts!

7.) *He will dote on his choice female.* He would long to get acquainted with your family members, following your 'guided' advice. He will be fluent, communicating with you in his love-languages. (My love languages are giving, serving, demonstrating and modeling purity, respect, and integrity). He would love to discover what your love languages are too.

8.) *He will brag of you to his friends – and will defend you before his family members to a fault!* If you experience any man dogging you out to his family, it's a tell-tale sign he will never marry you!

9.) *All men love the thoughts of sex. But a God-fearing man will set the tone of holiness unto the Lord – and his reverence of your body until after the wedding night before he would ask you for sex.* Even then, he doesn't just take it; he politely gives signals he's hungry for you. (A Godly man will not seduce you, sex-text or indulge in pornography).

10.) Lastly, he will so gloriously *intercede for you before the Lord!*

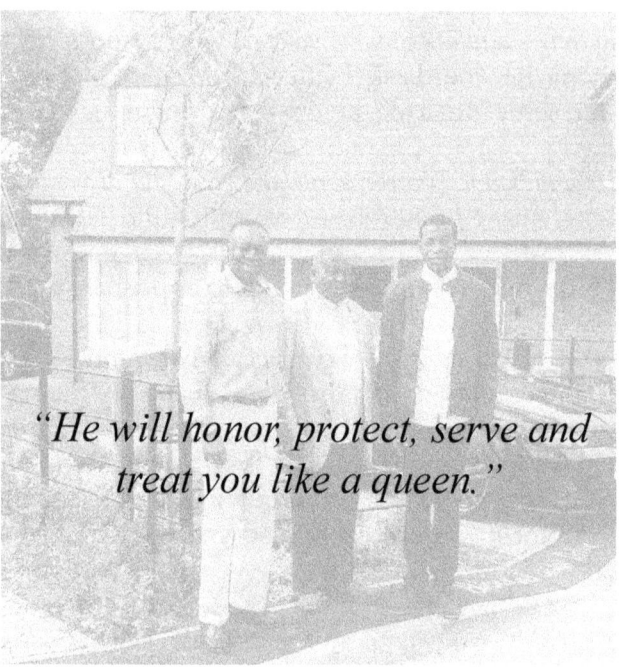

"He will honor, protect, serve and treat you like a queen."

In the oiriginal photo on page 98, Dr. Sammy Joseph models a genuine suitor paying a visit to his girlfriend's parent(s) and sibling. Courtesy, SJM, Birmingham, England. Copyrighted.

Lesson #37: Never Get Engaged without first Learning how to Harmoniously Resolve Your Disagreements!

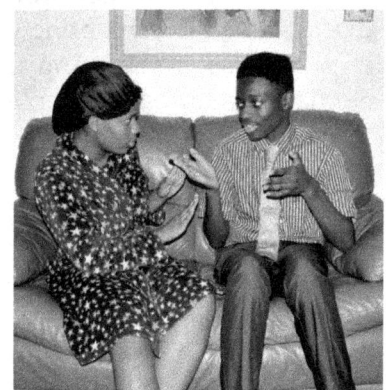

I

If all you've got going right now in your relationship is smooth *sailin'* with the one you intend to spend the rest of your life with, stop! Take a very deep breath, and recall when you did ever first have a major disagreement. Then recall how you had resolved or bridged that major rift. If you cannot recall any, the rule of the thumb from me to you is to *not* advance onto engagement so quickly! You may regret it.

Why?

Because we argue and disagree freely most, with people we feel at ease – and with whom we are most comfortable!

If your relationship is based on a *"Yes, yes, yes"* kind of a model, you're already a slave with a lost sense of identity and personality.

Even Father-God invites us to *"Come, let's reason together ..."* Isaiah 1:18. The key word here is "together." If your disagreement doesn't bring you more closely-knit together, what else would? And though you have an avowed eternal love for each other, spiritual-sense behooves you to take clues from "how" you've resolved past common disagreements:

• Did they start yelling like a child – or were they calm, and mature in handling matters?

• Did they offer a better insight to you now than you had, at the onset of the disagreement?

You need to know – and take special note! This is because, the very way they had treated you in a conflict-resolution season is the very same way you should expect to be treated when you've tied the knot with them. You would be surprised that in some marriages, some spouses had listened to – and sang way too much Craig David's *I'm Walkin' Away*, that they had not been able to differentiate reality from sheer musical lyrics when a storm had erupted in the tea-cup of their matrimony!

Let me give you an instance: A boy/girl-friend that broadcasts your hiccups to friends in your days of dating would certainly escalate to your very embarrassment, their broadcast to the entire world rife with a thousand-a-penny social media posts, about any trouble or trial in your marriage! Take that from me!

So, if you would avert un-necessary trouble and wounds of the soul, open your eyes, real wide! Wipe your face with a clean towel of reality. Love ain't blind, after all! No wise person trivializes the marriage covenant!

My job is to light your pathway with wisdom that will prevent possible future catastrophe in your marital union! I hope the intensity of this beam of light in this project hasn't left you dazzled and squinting!

"If your relationship is based on a "Yes, yes, yes" kind of a model, you're already a slave with a lost sense of identity and personality."

Original photo on the preceding page depicts a disagreeing, young couple definitely not disagreeable, courtesy SJM, Birmingham, England. Copyrighted.

Lesson #38: Getting Engaged? Never "Cut off" Your Parent(s).

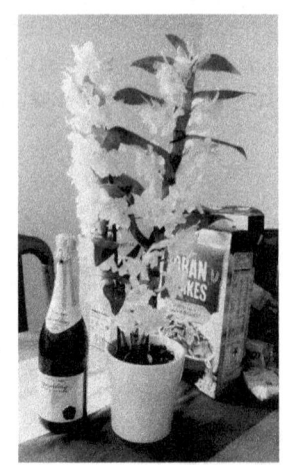

Not everyone emerged from 'solid', complete, traditional family units. A less-than-the-norm background should *not* define you.

Depending on your family make-up – or shake-up – do all in your power to introduce your parents to your promised future spouse. Now, I know I'm treading on a wet sand here. Nevertheless, nothing lesser than the wholesome truth should be expected to be communicated by me! After all, you didn't ask me for *an* opinion. You're kind enough to be reading my work: My sworn calling as a true minister of the Gospel forbids me from saying the unwholesome or partial truth.

As your servant-volunteer for the sake of Christ Jesus, therefore, I shall endeavor to enrich your life with what enriched experience of the past half a century of mine has yielded unto me. Remember, I have *not* advocated you involve all your family and extended family members in your matters. Let sleeping black sheep lie! I had said: *"Do all in your power to not cut off your parents"* because of a Godly reason I am about to intimate you with!

Even at my suggestion, let me make it crystal clear: Some parents are going to engage the 'rebuttal button' on their children's choices, offering them very contrary opinions. It's a huge pity that the young couple was caught unawares by the parent(s) trifling their love-life!

Some other times, it is one of the parents that will robustly withstand you. Particularly, if they are the controlling, narcissistic, gaslighting type! Some mothers still prefer to hold their children's imaginary umbilical cords wrapped around their arms. Some fathers will protest your plan as "just too sudden" – if you're a female – your erstwhile, joyful announcement of the introduction of your lover to him.

A divorced mother who had refused to *get a life* after her divorce may suddenly become jealous of her daughter – and her daughter's lover! Or become afraid of losing her son to her son's lover! Yet, some fathers would criticize and buck, citing "financial stress" as the reason for their butt-kicking aggravation at you – and/or your lover. These – and many more reactions are pieces of evidence of a parent's brokenness.

These fabricated excuses are both untenable – and unacceptable. Parents should be informed that they do *not* own their children/wards. Children are God's heritage. And both parents and grown adults should enjoy each other as God's institutional changes to life's varying seasons begin to transform their relationships. No one parent should constitute a hindrance to a son/daughter's God-given privilege of finding love and wanting to start their own family, the very right way of marriage!

If your family-scenario fits into any described above, wisdom authors me to advise you to be patient and *not* stubbornly rush ahead with your plans, to enforce your wish on – or over and above your parents'. Announcing your engagement and formal introductions to the family is the easier part. Planning the wedding ceremony to peacefully, reasonably accommodate the variables may be the harder part!

Try to not tribulate 'offending' parent(s). They may not have been there to perform their parental roles as you grew up. But wait; I say, they will forever be your biological parent(s). So let's agree to rightfully accord them their rights! Except they are incarcerated, have done outrageously or disowned you; accord parents the rights to meet your spouse-to-be and be present at your wedding! Most often times, if you're patient and prayerful, Father-God has ways of making obnoxious parents 'see reason' at the end of the day; winning their hearts over – and eventually supporting you both, spiritually, physically, financially and morally.

How long could you await obstinate parents' decision for, before you go ahead in your plans to marry?

I'd safely advise any time-lapse from between nine months to a year: It takes nine months to form and deliver a fully-developed baby. It couldn't take any more than a year to turn around a stiff neck!

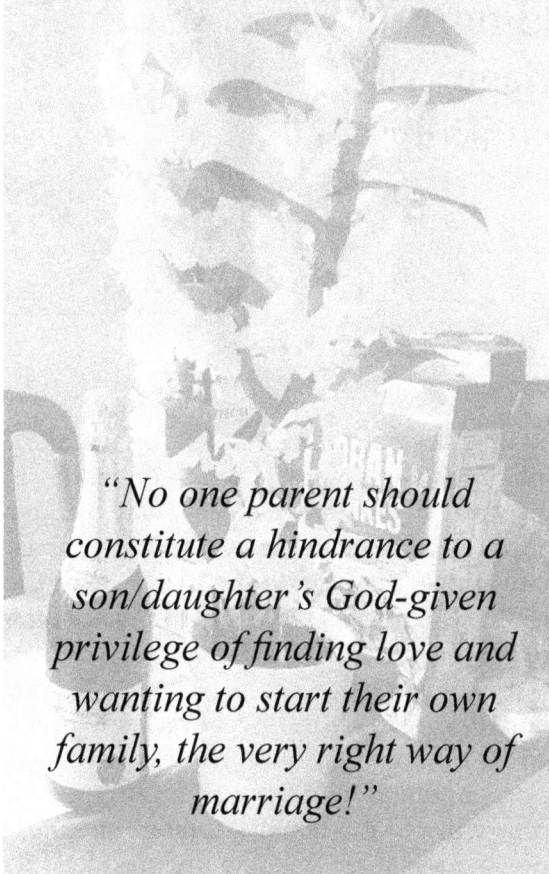

"No one parent should constitute a hindrance to a son/daughter's God-given privilege of finding love and wanting to start their own family, the very right way of marriage!"

Original photo: A white ichthus flower in a white vase, a bottle of wine – and boxes of cereal; SJM, Birmingham, England.Copyrighted.

Lesson #39: Wedding/ Marriage Preparations.

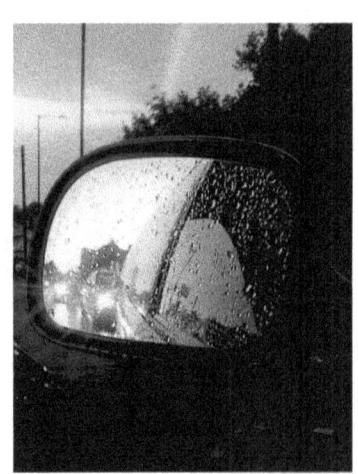

When planning for your wedding ceremony, by every possible means, avoid getting swept away by the wonderful emotions of a dance in the rain and the appearance of a rainbow above, that you forget to glance at the mirror of hindsight. The lessons hindsight offers are often found useful in perspective!

It's not out of place to see the lovebirds begin preparing for their marriage if they were wise. The less-wise-hearted will only be pre-occupied with the wedding-day preparations alone. You will see the females toning, tanning, weight-watching, gym-visiting, visiting the fashion designer's office many times for improvements and detail-changes inclusion. Their male counterparts are seen securing talks with employers for longer contract-renewals, paying frantic visits to the Estate agents and possibly, car-dealership shops. All these are good! However, the wisdom-driven spouse-to-be understands that a home is built on a little more than these afore-mentioned.

A home is built on the Wisdom of God – lest the builders build in vain. An intrinsic part of that wisdom is building within one's self, the beautiful, ornaments of a meek and quiet spirit; the fortification of the hidden human spirit with the grace of God! That grace corrects in perspective, the defective backgrounds of the spouses-to-be while making gains on already solidified contexts!

Never wed anyone without first, placing under the microscopic spotlight of the gracious Holy Spirit, the defective backgrounds of both yours and your partner's!

> *"Never wed/marry without first, placing under the microscopic spotlight of the gracious Holy Spirit, the defective backgrounds of both yours and your partner!"*

Original copyrighted photo courtesy of GabbyStudio, Lancaster, England.
A greyscale picture of a rainy twilight as seen through the side driving mirror of a car overlooking a beautiful rainbow on the horizon.
(Can you sight the rainbow?)

Lesson #40: Marriage!

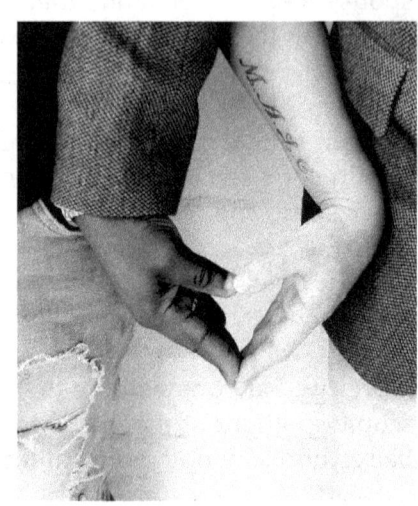

How could anyone teach about marriage in three or four paragraphs of writing? That is such an impossible task! However, if you look very carefully when couples touch the tips of their fingers bent sideways, what shape they form is that of a heart, ♥ – the shape of love! And right above the love sign is the shape of a diamond! A couple holding hands, however, do achieve far much more than forming a mere signage. Their act of holding hands puts them in remembrance of their vows: *"To hold and cherish in sickness and in health, for richer or poorer, 'till death does us part!"*

No human can fully comprehend the love of God – for God is Love! And the marriage institution – between a husband and a wife – is meant to be the exact replica of his love for us!

Love teaches the couple *how* they are meant to live the rest of their days together, that is, united in love as one! They two are one, valued, protected; a precious item of far more worth than mere gold! That is the golden rule of the thumb: A husband's willingness to lay down his life for his wife. And the wife in return, honoring and respecting her husband without inhibition or restraints. By so doing, they both would be protecting, valuing, esteeming, honoring, preserving, and cherishing each other as valued jewels of inestimable worth before the Lord!

Should any married couple pursue these virtues – with an added immeasurable dosage of the ingredient called forgiveness – no power in hell could ever conquer their love! Any surprising, masking upheaval that rears up its ugly head against that union would be very well swallowed up by the quality of life of that marriage!

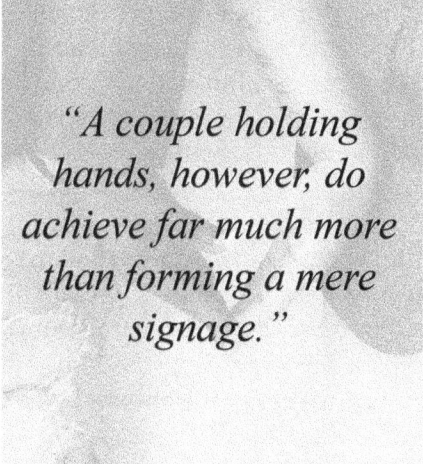

"A couple holding hands, however, do achieve far much more than forming a mere signage."

Original photo on the preceding page shows a couple forming the symbols of a heart – and a diamond; courtesy, SJM, Birmingham, England. Copyrighted.

Lesson #41: The Gift of Sex and Sexuality.

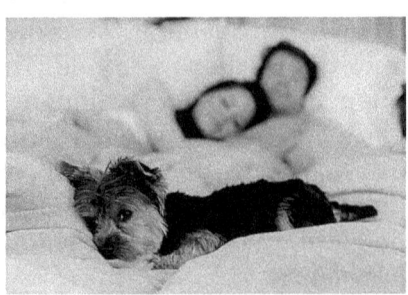

Notice how I have described this *very* topic: *"The Gift of Sex and Sexuality,"* for it is a gift; first, from the Creator to us humans. Every male and female inhabiting this planet, Earth, possesses this gift. But *not* everyone knows how to contain, release, use and share their sexuality with another!

This free gift endowed us by the Creator, some have converted into the wickedest weapon of collateral, emotional damage basically because of their lack of judgment. Or because they probably have been misinformed, misled, misguided or abused regarding the honorable safe-keep of the voracious appetite of the animal instincts within!

Widen your eyebrow at me if you may, at my erstwhile informing that you possess 'animal instincts' deep within; but nothing could be farther from the truth if you are wrapped up in a fuzzy kind of blanket of denial of same! This instinct – aided by hormones secreted into the bloodstream – helps couples consummate their holy matrimonies! It is also that aggression-causing, jealousy-arousing feeling (basically for the sole reason of territorial protection for safe-keep and wellness), flowing in the veins of a spouse towards the other. This protectionist instinct was not sinful in its original intent!

Your sexuality is yours. That remains true for every unmarried/single person. God expects you to master it well – so that you would indeed rightly contain, release, use, and share it when the rightful occasion calls upon you to do so.

However, if you're married – as you probably would have found out anyway, your sexuality *no longer* remains exclusively yours for the keeps! Just like every other gift or mess you brought with you into that marriage/relationship; femininity, and her curvaceousness must *not* now be deployed by the wife/(female) as a tool for supremacy and manipulation of the male. Neither should the husband's/(male) sturdy masculinity, six-pack tummy ripples or turgid manhood be deployed as instruments of subjugation, control or a reign of terror over the female companion! I say this because the matters of unbridled, uncontrolled, un-sanctimonious sex and sexuality are the very first after money-matters raised in counseling, by quarreling couples. Unfaithfulness, revenge-affairs, withholding sex as punishment *etcetera* are rampant destroyers too – even in many a Christian marriage! This unbridled tongue of flesh between the limbs of dispassionate men and women have led to many horrific sex-crimes, domestic violence cases, separation/divorces, homicides, and suicides!

At all times, open, honest, sincerest communication, consideration for one's spouse, coupled with a maximum dosage of self-control are the three most beautiful, most romantic virtues a wedded couple could possess when reality dawns on their sexuality. The engagement of these will further enrich their sexual union – including any other need(s) their marital and sexual lives may have!

And please, could you kindly keep cats, dogs, bunnies – and other pets, including your much beloved little babies and toddlers away from your romantic bed always?

(Obtain my book: 'APPRECIABLE Gifts' from *harvestways. org* – or anywhere books are sold online for in-depth discussions on your relationships, marriage, and sexuality. This book also contains other suggested authors' titles that should help you satisfy your quests – as it had, countless others!)

"If you're married – as you probably would have found out anyway, your sexuality no longer remains entirely, exclusively yours for the keeps!"

The picture of a couple in bed with their dog. (Accessed https://media.mnn.com/assets/images/2015/10/couple-bed-dog.jpg.838x0_q80.jpg October 16, 2018 at 22:43 Hrs.)

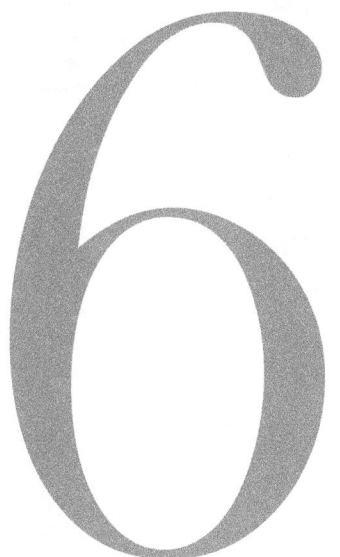

PART SIX

Unhealthy Marriage, Counseling, Separation, Divorce – And Co-Habitation

Lesson #42: Unhealthy Marriage, Counseling, Separation, Divorce – and Cohabitation.

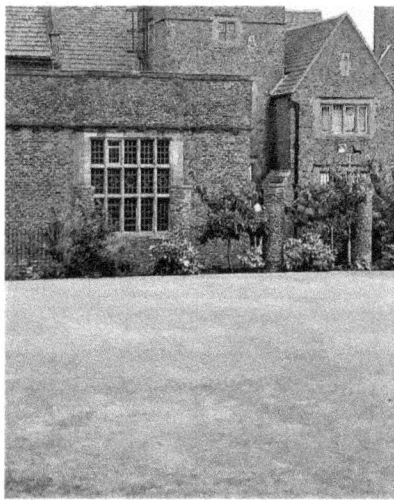

I confirm there are many unhealthy marriages – just as there are unhealthy souls. I have seen – and at times mediated in far more than could be counted off my finger-tips! Some counseling sessions had led to a re-think, a soul-search between the couples for healing and miraculous restorations! Some others, I am afraid, had led to weariness; a wear-and-tear of the spirit because of the underlying decay and rottenness like the decay embedded in a tooth's root-canal, whenever *either* of the parties had refused to fully submit their *dentition* for cleaning and waxing!

An Unhealthy Marriage

I define an unhealthy marriage as one in which one or more guidelines surrounding the sustainability of a biblical marriage relationship has been broken. A marriage wherein abounds abuse, domestic violence, and various unquantifiable violations. I have always been an unbridled, express, advocate for a divorce-petition at the Court *if* it could be demonstrated beyond doubts that there was – or had ever been an abuse, or a violation suffered by either a spouse and/or the children who are minors in the marriage!

Separation and Divorce

As you probably do know, a divorce cannot be effected until it has been demonstrated to a Judge that the petitioned ground(s) for the dissolution of that marriage is/are indeed, undeniably proven beyond reasonable conclusions! Most often, a divorcing couple will undergo a period of remorse, followed by bitterness, a tantrum-spell, a brokenness or a revengeful vendetta-plan. Any of these could lead to the death of one – and/or the suicide of the other! Anyone – along with the children – undergoing a toxic circumstance ought to be automatically granted an urgent separation from their surviving spouse before an impending, imploding tragedy occurs!

Granted, Father-God hates both separation and divorce. But so also does He equally hate dysfunctional relationships/marriages as I have earlier mentioned.

He possibly couldn't hate more, both the confusion and the hatred of hearts that always ensue when divorced, ex-partners co-habit under the same roof!

Unhealthy Marriage, Counseling, Separation, Divorce – and Co-Habitation

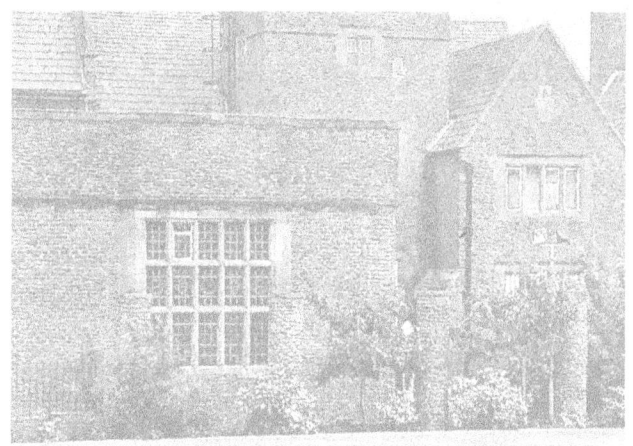

"An unhealthy marriage as one in which one or more guidelines surrounding the sustainability of a biblical marriage relationship has been broken!"

Original photo is of a beautiful, Brewer's Tudor-styled cottage built in Cotswold stone enclosed by a lush, terraced back garden; SJM, Birmingham, England. Copyrighted.

Lesson #43: Cohabiting Ex-spouses.

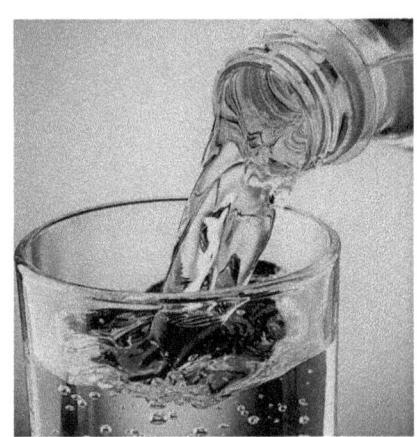

Every human whose inner organs are working at *par* – or above *par* – experiences a thirst/hunger-pang. It is as natural an inclination to physical hunger as it is to sexual hunger! But wait: Sex is *not* included on the list of physiological needs like air to breathe, food to eat and clothe to wear to keep the body warm. Those are the major, essential needs every human *must* have in order to stay alive!

Now, ex-spouses who cohabit do so for various reasons under the sun. The main reason always is financial constraints *"splitting the equity in the house that has not sold."* But I have understudied enough cohabiting ex-couples, to realize that there are more reasons than just the locked-up equity in the house that keeps them glued together still, in their co-opted lifestyle! Some just can't let go of the lure of *"the strong sex bond we shared!"* So, they keep warming up in-between the sheets because of unprepared-for bouts of loneliness and the ensuing depression that have suddenly accosted them. Some others cite the need for co-parenting as the reason while they still live under the same roof while bringing in different, new lovers into the very same abode.

These are abominable, abhorrent, costly practices! Somebody needs to apply some discretion here – and stop the madness even if the male needs to domicile in the car, in the public park, until he finds himself another suitable roof! And may I say that not all divorcees are frivolous. So, on their behalf, I ask that you please be sensitive. And to those of you who would love to be obstinate, I humbly ask that you keep your suspicions to yourself! Not everyone who had divorced had wanted to be divorced!

That above was an actual lesson that had dawned upon my understanding with age and experience: Some had *had* divorce forced upon them by circumstances beyond their control. Some had never loved the spouse they had forcibly been culturally subjected to, marrying, through arranged marriages! Others had married at immature ages just to escape troubles at home. And others more had married, as a means of pacifying their stupid, irrational, uncontrollable, passionate desires!

I had been forced to separate at first, from my wife of eight years in 2004 due to the violent, mental and domestic violations I had suffered in the marriage. More importantly, I knew God would hold me responsible for having the power - to shield from harm my life, and my five, little children - but had failed to exercise that power, had I died in the violence meted out to me. He would have found me culpable of six, 'first-degree' murders brought on by my sheer negligence!

After I had been thoroughly violated, bruised, and bloody-beaten, she would dial *999* directed to the Police. In those dark days of British policing, the Force had presumed the male as always the aggressor – and had proceeded to make an arrest of him.

I had been arrested and locked up in un-dignified Police cell holdings overnight, for a totality of twenty-one hours on a couple of occasions, barely ten months apart. With no criminal record ever traceable to me, the Law had *had* to let go of me! But the innocent children had been exposed to an unprecedented risk of being snatched upon by the State – and fostered across the entire topography of the United Kingdom with new names and identities! That imminent threat I had to assassinate!

So, someday, at another altercation involving her choke-hold on my neck wherein I had hardly been able to breathe; as soon as I had struggled to break free of her strangulation attempt on me, I had thought to myself, just one word: "Enough!" That same day, I had called the Police! The process of ending the unhealthy marriage had commenced. Legal paperwork had been filed – alongside the gory, photographic pieces of evidence from a decade of abuse. I had asked for a Protective Order alongside a divorce! Originally, my intention had been to serve her a rude awakening of a loud, ringing, wake-up bell; peradventure God will grant her the grace to confront herself. But no; she had continued with her secret escapades with different men while the divorce had not even been pronounced. She had indeed re-married shortly, thereafter!

She would later engage me in a four-and-a-half-year-long, child custody battle, at the Family Courts. The eldest child had just turned seven at the time – and the other two sets

Unhealthy Marriage, Counseling, Separation, Divorce – and Co-Habitation

of twins had all been well below four years old, and in diapers! At the end of this grueling tenure, the Judge had granted me full custody of the children – and had placed a restraining order upon her to never have further physical contact with any of them until they were adults, except via mail correspondence alone, with no compliant force whatsoever laid upon any child to reply!

In spite of my testimony, may I humbly submit to you: There's never a winner in a divorce situation! The job of a twin-engine, cargo plane, with a shut-down engine would always bear far-reaching consequences, except for the undeniable grace of God. A word, is I think, is enough for the consideration of the wise!

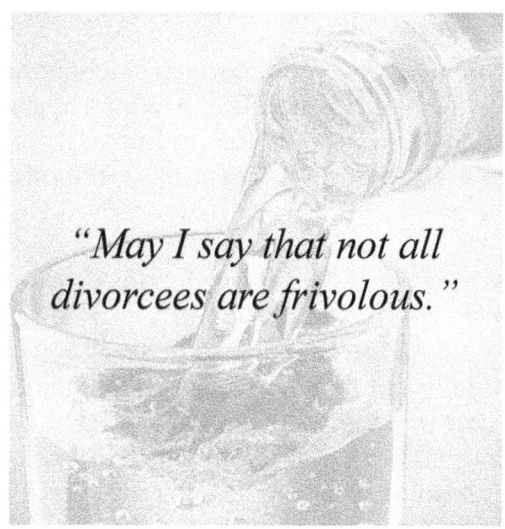

"May I say that not all divorcees are frivolous."

Original photo of page 120 shows a cup of cold, carbonated water from the refrigerator.
Courtesy, SJM, Birmingham, England.

Lesson #44: Life after Divorce.

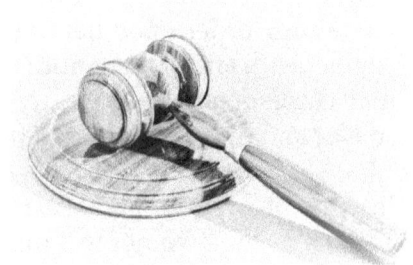

I suppose many factors militate against a holy matrimony than meets the natural eyes. That is why a husband and a wife must always intercede for, and protect each other – and their family, under the covering of the impenetrable Lamb's Blood.

But if your marriage had been dissolved, I am sorry to learn of that unfortunate situation!

To remain holy unto the Lord, a separated spouse cannot possibly start looking for new love while still being married. Doing so is termed an affair; which technically speaking, is wholesome adultery. Having an affair is the next most abhorrent practice to the holy God, after idolatry!

Legal rudiments require married parties attend mediation many times before a divorce case could be heard before a

Family Judge. Counseling too may be recommended, *if* the legal experts deem the marriage as redemptive. That clearly depicts to anyone that *not* every divorce case is the same. In fact, aggravated couples who bring up the matter of divorce as the only available option instead of first communicating with each other with a view to settling their differences, are unethical. Selfish spouses who are hell-bent on having their selfishness imposed upon their spouses and the entire family must be blighted with some undiagnosed, mental, neuro-misfirings and misjudgments!

I have counseled couples who state, flatly: *"I have fallen out love with him/her."* I think, simply put, that is plain demonic – and callous. No one can fall out of love and live! Remember, God is love! What these have experienced is a different season of love which they are ill-equipped for, and most unprepared to handle; one which they simply have refused to grow into!

If you 'fell out' of love, experienced a divorce – and are conjoined by children, may I lovingly warn you to tread softly? Divorce involving child(ren) will always be tough. I know there are some nasty spouses – particularly wives/females who fabricate lies and serious allegations against their children's fathers. They 'coach' the young daughters to allege a sexual misconduct, an abuse, or a sexual impropriety against their fathers when indeed nothing of such had occurred. Listen to my conclusive summary of you: You are sick and complicatedly pathetic!

Divorced people by law *may* legally re-marry, by the laws of man; yet, God hates both separation – and the actual divorce | *Malachi 2:14-16*. But again, I say, He also hates all manner of abuse – and violence! Frivolities and trifling with marriage-vows are also an abhorrence to Him!

Choosing A New Partner

I am unable to say, to what extent your jurisdiction and yardstick-parameters are, for choosing a new partner. Or whether you may re-marry as a divorcee! You would need to settle that with your God – and your conscience!

But I could offer you some guidelines if asked. Should you want to request my guidelines on the topic we have been talking about, please ask for my book *APPRECIABLE Gifts* from *harvestways.org* – or anywhere books are sold online. Should you love to book a counseling session with me, then kindly e-mail at *'admin@harvestways.org'*

Except the Lord Himself brings you a partner that is so angelic that he/she would indeed emotionally adopt love for your child(ren) – particularly minor children, I would propose that you be considerate enough to allow those child(ren) to mature to become full adults first, before you advance onto considering re-marrying! This may sound harsh, but there's great wisdom in practicing deferred gratification, for the survivability of your young ones!

Whatever you choose to do, just don't put *any* stranger in there with your child/ward. Did you hear me loud and clear? Don't bring a monster home to your child/ward!

Remove that Divorcee Name-tag; Please!

Some divorcees never could recover from the divorce ordeal. More than a few divorced persons would willingly agree to put up with those evil name tags normally labeled, ready for divorcees. They proudly wear and refer to them in every of their life's conversations!

It doesn't have to necessarily be that way, my friend! You

may choose to be single to serve the Lord for the rest of your days. Happily serving younger couples/persons in pre-marital counseling could be a tremendously rewarding, beautiful ministry!

You may choose to start, run or fund an orphanage. And if older, possibly focus on your grand-children to help watch and raise them. Or you may join your church's/ministry's outreach, volunteer at events, or engage in other worthy, charitable activities! Just ensure that you do *not* occupy an empty, lonely, dark house, feeling sorry or pity for yourself!

Never allow the guilt-feeling for wrong, past decisions or sins God has no record of to rent a space upstairs above your neck!

I hope I am well understood?

"If you 'fell out' of love, experienced a divorce – and are conjoined by children, may I lovingly warn you to tread softly?"

Photo of a Family Judge's gavel. Courtesy SJM, Birmingham, England.

PART SEVEN

Raising Godly Children

Lesson #45:
Show God to Your Children Early in Life.

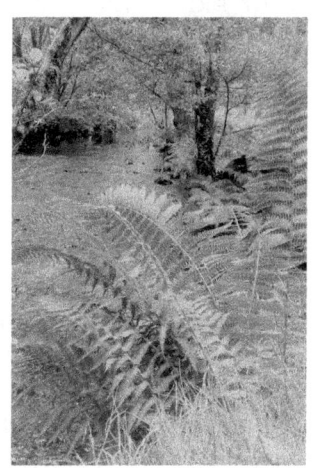

King David mentioned such restorative blessedness of a restorative brook of water where the Lord is the Shepherd. Such had been what Father-God had originally designed family-units to be: Brooks of *"still waters"* | *Psalms 23:2*.

By God's special grace alone, I have – as a single parent – successfully raised five, loving, God-honoring, young adults. Admittedly, I grew spurious, sliver-linings raising those five; but you know, I also thrived in the process! When people ask me: *How did you manage to do that?* My response always is: *"God Almighty helped me with His tremendous anointing!"*

God enabled me to encounter Him early! With that great gift of a personal encounter with the Lord Jesus at the tender age of three, I was able to introduce Him to others – starting first, with my immediate family!

That's the very same thing you've got to do: Create for your kids ample opportunities to have a first-hand encounter with the Lord, Jesus, early! Gently lead them by the meadows of quietness and peace.

How early is "early"?

"Early" is as early as you both discover you're expecting a child in the womb!

Little children's minds are very soft and tender. Hearts are best molded when young! So, seize the advantages youth, innocence and fun offer you. Use these prayerfully as effective tools. Read Godly books to them to expand their minds. Watch Godly television shows/DVD's together. Listen to their inquisitive minds – and encourage them to learn by heart, worship songs, and scriptural portions. Answer their questions with appropriate, truthful, Biblical stories. Create and color together, pictorial books with insightful memories. Keep a stack of digital pictures and videos, documenting their growth – and life's journeys. Keep those children shielded away from corrupting influences – and individuals!

Allow them to have their own friends. Owing to my personal convictions, I never did allow any of my children a 'sleep-over' at any of their friends'. None of those parents had been born-again Christians!

Divorced, separated or foster-parents shouldn't dull their child's/ward's sunshine. Always separate the child from your ex-spouse. You cannot afford to badmouth your spouse/ex-spouse to the child. That would be emotionally damaging to them. You must not reveal 'damaging facts' about the other parent to them, either. That would wreak havoc. A statement such as: *"You cannot trust her; she tried to abort your pregnancy,"* is an unmanly, un-stately, and an uncalled-for, line of thought! It will incense a child to hostility and hatred for the mother – and all who had encouraged that pregnancy to be aborted.

Never say I never warned you!

Just rather raise the children rightly, regardless of whatever circumstance(s) you may be enduring, have endured – or will endure! Let go. And let God!

If you did raise the child well, you have the re-assuring promise of God that they will *not* depart from the Way of Righteousness shown them when they've grown older and wiser | *Proverbs 23:7*.

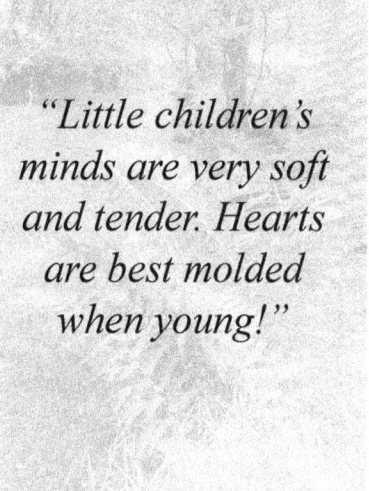

"Little children's minds are very soft and tender. Hearts are best molded when young!"

Original photo: A serene, calm atmosphere of a meadow in Snowdonia, Wales, United Kingdom.
Courtesy GabbyStudio, Lancaster, England. Copyrighted.

Lesson #46: Always Apply the 'Fair-play' Rule to the Child.

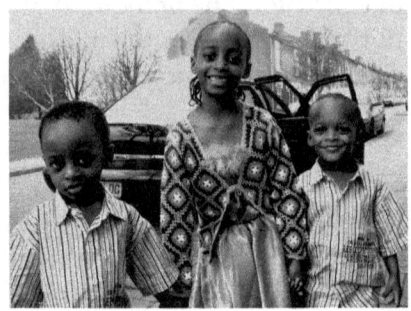

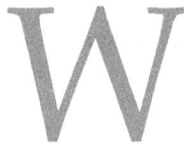

When I trained as a classroom teacher at the University of Warwick in England for my Post Graduate studies in 2003, one of the lessons drummed into our cohort was: *"Always apply to the child, the fair-play rule!"*

What then was the teacher's 'fair-play rule'?

> *The 'fair-play rule' stipulated that the teacher must always be fair to the child, reward the child for every good behavior – and sanction appropriately, his/her bad behavior. While applying the sanction to a child, the teacher must ensure the child understands the reason why he/she was being sanctioned!*

Every child knows both the thrill and the importance to his/her ego, an award brings. But not everyone – not excluding even you, an adult – appreciates the majestic clamping down of the law upon them in punitive sanctions even when the reasons have been made crystal clear! Such is the precept upon which the Prison systems of the world were formed!

A child disciplined in love and great understanding with firmness while young, will more than likely respond to the rationale behind the chastening – and become a responsible adult!

Do *not* laugh at a child under discipline. That's is not the application of the 'fair-play-rule'! That is simply cruel. Someday, that child will become an adult – who never forgot the parent's cruel remarks, laughter or mockery at a time you may have become too old to even recall!

Be *very* dutiful to your kids/wards. Be careful in exercising power, authority, and restraints to a stubborn young child! Do not break their spirit while training them!

If you're raising more than a child, be unequivocally clear to them, they are *all* equally important – with no one as your favorite! Only say what you mean and mean what you say to a child! Children are quick to perceive adult insecurities and lies. Don't you ever let a child label you a liar!

Never let a child manipulate you against your spouse/partner. And, do not neglect your child/ward. Exposing your child/ward to the risks of being abused by anyone is a chargeable child-neglect offense for which you may rightly so lose that child to the State! Above all, balance work and play with your child/ward – and family.

Forgive him/her easily.

Humble yourself before the innocent spirit of any that you have wronged. Apologize, kneeling before him/her as you would have begged for mercy from an adult if you had to. (I had assumed the kneeling position before my children a few times as I'd wrongly disciplined the innocent one! That was yet another significant part of the "fair-play rule" I had learned as a parent!)

"A child disciplined in love and great understanding with firmness while young, will more than likely respond to the rationale behind the chastening – and become a responsible adult!"

Photo of the first three siblings in the Joseph household: Gabby in the middle, flanked by twin brothers, Dan and Dave in 2003. Courtesy Sammy Joseph Ministries, Birmingham, England.

Lesson #47: Money-matter and Strong Work Ethics.

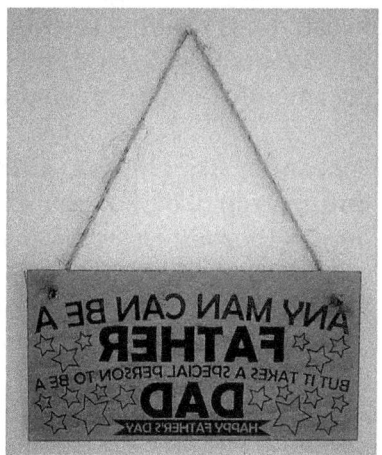

I received this wall decor from my quiver-set, some time ago. It still hangs above my head at our dining table. Now, if you could read its message without blinking, you would be eligible for a strong 'Pass' in the money-matter/financial discipline talks we had held at that table!

The truth is, financial education is *not* included in the formal education years of your youngster. No one models before the *younglings*, lessons involving financial management, discipline – and credit control.

Up until today, I do *not* have a credit card anywhere in the world!

I modeled before my little ones early, the importance of strong, dedicated work ethics, astute financial management, a saving mentality and a heavy-investment culture of sowing into the Kingdom of God. I raised them up living moderately frugal. I did not purchase anything on a loan. I cut my coat according to my size. I did not bite much more than I could chew even if that meant purchasing smooth-running, second-hand, vehicles!

Whenever an enticing Credit Card application flew through our letterbox-doorpost, the young adults knew how to chorus: *"Here comes our enemy, Dad!"*

Not until they had fully become reasonable, well-reined adults had I called and sat them down to explain to them that owning a credit card is *"not entirely wrong if you could repay the amount spent on capital purchases days before the month-end interest rate is applied."* One of them had sighed at that de-briefing! You should have seen the faces of the others!

This should make you either glad or sad: It's the work ethics your children know you by that they too will reproduce in their adult years!

> *"The truth is, financial education is not included in the formal education years of your youngster."*

Photo: A significant component of Dr. Sammy Joseph's 2017 Fathers' Day gift from his children. Courtesy SJM, Birmingham, England.

Lesson #48: When Children Leave Home.

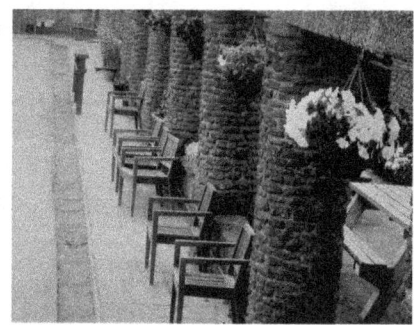

Take it from me: Your children will grow and leave home, someday! Your evening sun-gazing chairs will soon become empty! *"It always happens so very quickly."* So, do parents say! Between the time you first cuddled each of them in your arms and the very day you loaded their stuff into the trunk/booth of the car – and chauffeured them to their University halls of residence, the time is unbelievable short! This transition could be very traumatic for some parents! Then comes the parting hugs. And if you're the teary type, the tears!

They have clocked eighteen, the age of full, legal accountability! You arrived at their residence with a fully loaded car. Now, you *will* return home, empty. (Except probably with your spouse – if you're married or have a partner). It is a new season of life. It announces to you: Growth and Continuum!

What blessedness!

Yet emotions rule the day – and will possibly, for many more weeks or months!

If you're a Godly parent, you would release your young adult child/ward to grow and flourish. To gracefully emerge from beneath your shadows, discover him/herself *en route* becoming a healthy individual!

First, I refuse to use the term "empty-nester parents" because Scripture says your quiver is full! Your quiver is no fuller because you have a larger number of children/wards than that of the parents of a lone child! God's criterion for rewards, Jesus says, are in categories of *"thirty-fold, sixty-fold and a hundred-fold"* | Matthew 13:8.

Second, you're moving along just fine in God's timetable. If you have raised your child/ward well – as I have earlier described, you are not apprehensive about the kind of adults they would emerge into.

I have experienced far too many children who couldn't wait to "turn legal" before they had turned on their parents attacking them through various means and styles. This is one irrefutable proof of either a horrible parenting for two decades, or a child-personality disorder. The young adult shouts down at their parents. These get rude – and become forceful. Some even snarl and snap at them, invading their personal spaces. All the suppressed pains of the past fifteen years surge to the surface like a huge tidal *tsunami* wave. The atmosphere is electric. Someone *must* de-escalate the tense, hostile atmosphere, by leaving the scene, room or house!

Be assured: All hopes of peace are not lost.

Fruits are always bigger than seeds!

Righteousness will yet prevail in your relationship with your young adult. But you must relate that his/her sails are no more in your hands – but in God's! And you must hands-off, totally to Him!

While an aggravated parent can *possibly* do nothing to acquiesce a raging, youthful, adult child, you can still moor his/her tentacles to the Everlasting Arms. Father-God will surely deliver and restore double, that which the cankerworms, locusts, and palmerworms had eaten. That is His everlasting promise.

Keep your tongue busy declaring peace over your children and posterity in Jesus name – and your declarations shall come to pass, most assuredly.

Never wait until your child/ward has left home before you had started to intercede for him/her about their future, choices of a spouse, career, settlement-locations *etcetera*. Parents mold their children's lives from the womb by intercessory prayers, until the day that they precede them in death!

Avoid calamities; don't be caught napping, prayerless! That could be much costlier than any could dare pay!

"While an aggravated parent can possibly do nothing to acquiesce a raging, youthful, adult child, you can still moor his/her tentacles to the Everlasting Arms."

Original photo: A pretty bouquet of flower-baskets hanging on Cotswold-stone pillars at a public place; courtesy, SJM, Birmingham, England.

Part Eight

Healthy Foods/Drinks Choices

Lesson #49: Eat Greaseless, Healthy Meals!

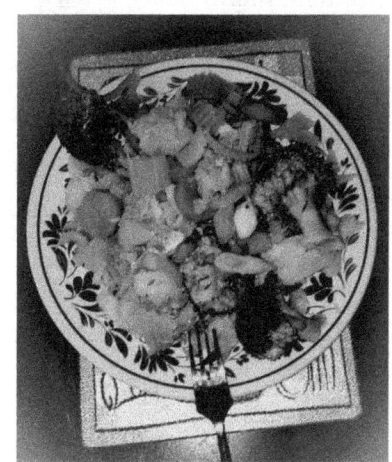

Here's the photograph of my late breakfast/brunch meal this beautiful Wednesday: Some Alaskan Pollock, broccoli, carrots, ginger, garlic, and celery. (Some other days, I prefer turkey or chicken breast to fish). These would all be well washed down – with two glasses of clean, lemon-infused water!

I'm *not* too adept at teaching how to eat healthily – but I sure will share with you the practical knowledge that the Lord has allowed me to successfully acquire over time! I won't hold a thing back! That I had promised at the opening of this book – and that I shall disclose in the closing section of this book!

(And oh; by the way, I stopped using a knife as part of my cutlery a year ago this day – and a spoon, two years previous! Let's see what next will be axed from my graceful table manners this year!)

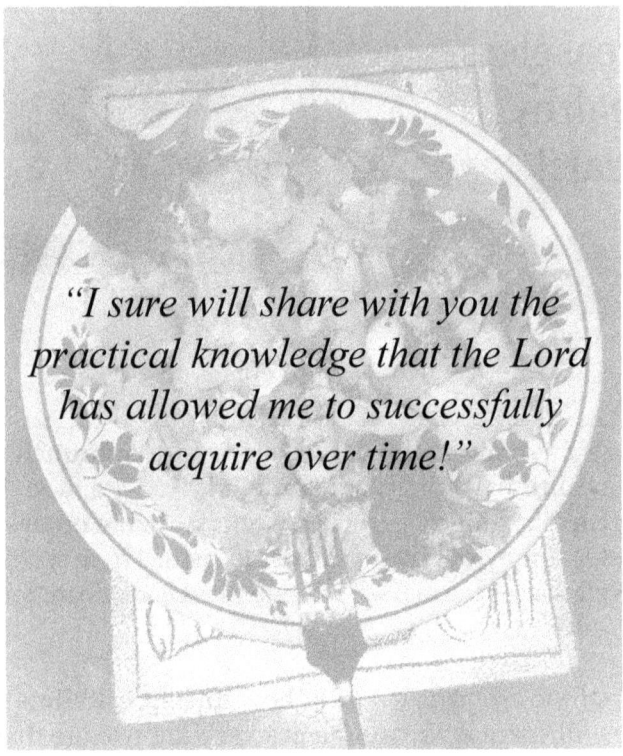

"*I sure will share with you the practical knowledge that the Lord has allowed me to successfully acquire over time!*"

Photo of Dr. Sammy Joseph's plate of a healthy, late breakfast/brunch meal. Copyrighted, SJM, Birmingham, England.

Lesson #50: Drink Healthy, Costless, Home-made Drinks.

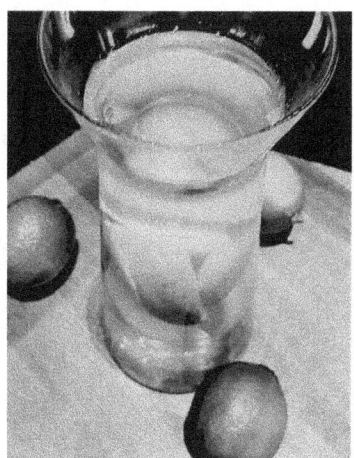

Lemon sliced in warm or cold water (based on preference), helps detoxify the skin, the body – and the internal organs. This inexpensive drink can become a substitute for artificially sweetened orange/apple/juice-drinks that are detrimentally high in sugar content!

Lemon-infused water-drink did indeed help me shed some unwanted weight within a relatively short period of three months. I had suddenly noticed I had shrunk from 85kg/187lbs to 72kg/158lbs. I had lost six inches off my waistline without any effort whatsoever different to subtracting sugar or sugary drinks from my intake. That ought to be good news to anyone who wants to shrink their excess flesh.

Depending upon your desired weight, you could add body-building exercises to your regiment to tighten the muscles in your body – and that also would be healthy.

Lemon-infused water also has a high concentrate of Vitamin C – and aids digestion!

Try a cup a day, starting today!

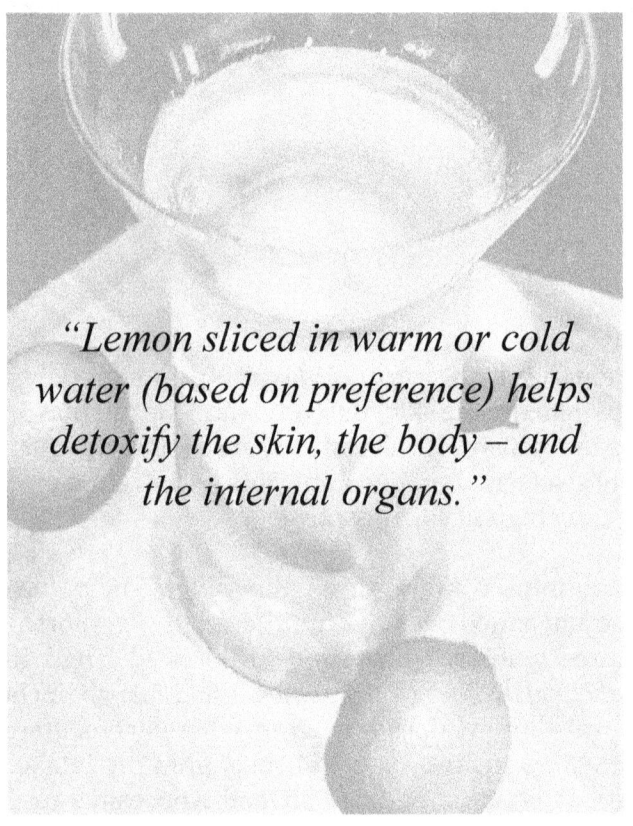

"Lemon sliced in warm or cold water (based on preference) helps detoxify the skin, the body – and the internal organs."

Photo: A jug of cold, lemon-infused refreshing water ready to be served as a detoxifying drink courtesy SJM, Birmingham, England.

PART NINE

Extras on Health & Fitness; And Healthy Lifestyle Choices

#1: The Best Healthy Food of All Times: The Bible.

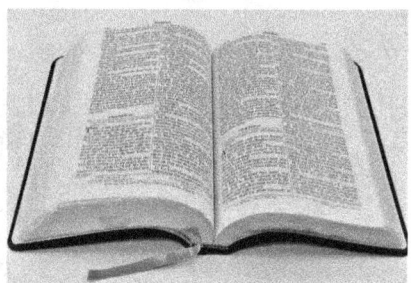

G

God's Word is sweeter than the honeycomb. It is to be desired than a daily meal ration. This is the Holy Bible. The words on these pages become health to your navel as you read. A chapter-a-day reading or listening habit on the new apps, is like a health capsule taken: It keeps both spiritual and physical diseases at bay!

A chapter in the daytime – and another read before bedtime will detoxify your soul from the day's routine – and soar you above demonic principalities and powers! I enjoy reading the Bible. I love the stories and the Prophets. I love the parables and the teachings of Jesus, but most of all, I love the Pauline letters. The psalms and observations of Job and King Solomon are magnificent.

Let me encourage you to be a soul-fit, Spirit-fed human being, by asking you to start cultivating the habit of a daily, Bible-reading/listening schedule! You will not *regret* it!

#2: Eat Healthy, Home-cooked foods.

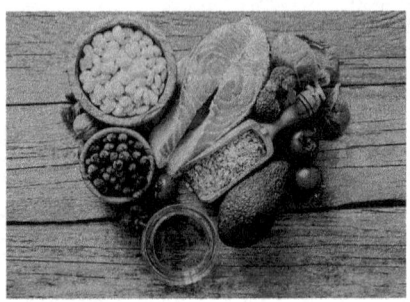

The food choices in the picture above include an avocado, salmon fish – in fact, for my taste buds, any non-fatty fish is great – blueberries, dried natural nuts, ground herbs and vegetables like tomatoes, broccoli, spinach *etcetera*.

Here are a few of my suggestions for your daily ration:

1.) Consume more variant fruit-types and vegetables, daily.

2.) Drastically reduce your intake of bread, rice, pasta – and *all* starchy foods. If you must eat bread, eat whole grain, wheat bread and cereals – in moderation.

3.) Go 'green' – or if you like, 'vegan': Eat healthy, green, leafy shoots – for instance, cabbage, lettuce, spinach and kale, collard green, spring green; Brussel sprouts, radishes, and legumes such as beans, peas, *etcetera*.

4.) Go 'nutty'; that is, snack on natural nuts – and not packed snacks.

5.) Substitute oily fish and skinless poultry for most red meat.

6.) Enjoy two to three servings of low-fat or fat-free dairy choices twice or thrice a week, such as a glass of milk, yogurt, or low-fat cheese.

7.) Above all, incorporate consistent exercise regimes into your weekly routine; possibly lasting at least three, half-hour sessions, spread throughout the week!

#3: Eat Bitter Melons.

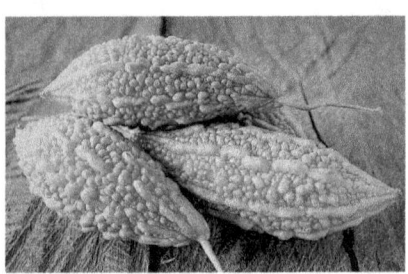

On my social media platforms in March 2018, I had posted a whole month of healthy foods, drink – and lifestyle choices; you may want to search my name on there and read!

The picture above is that of bitter melons. Bitter melons may prove elusive in England due to their seasonal availability. Hence, they could be a highly priced fruit. (One sure way to beat the departmental stores at overcharging you, is to call your city's council and inquire about the availability of its Farmers'/Wholesale Market. They should be able to inform you of its availability/non-availability and opening times).

Bitter melons are perfect for balancing or reducing the high glucose/sugar levels in the blood. They are a huge booster to your health and wellbeing!

#4: Snack on Dried Nuts.

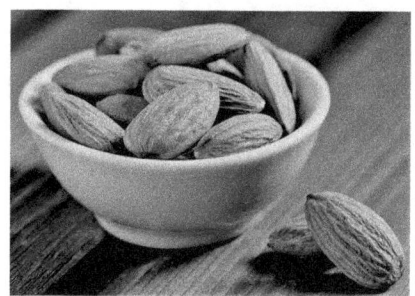

Isn't it of great observation to note that the Patriarch Jacob did not send the sneaky, appealing, tempting, chocolatey *Mars Bars* and cakes of Canaan to Joseph as presents in Egypt? Instead, he asked his sons to pack *"the best fruits in the land"* | Genesis 43:11. And when they did, kindly take special notice of the fruits instructed: *Natural honey, some balsamic spices, almonds and pistachio nuts.*

Moderate honey is a substitute for processed white sugar – an artificial killer!

Balsam is aromatic. It can also can be used to treat hemorrhoids, tumors, heart and chest-pains – and also, all inflammations.

Pistachios are healthy antioxidants useful for lowering cholesterol, blood sugar – and improving the eye and blood vessel health.

Lastly, almonds help sharpen brain activities, prevent heart attacks and control blood sugar among other benefits!

#5: Say 'No' to Donuts.

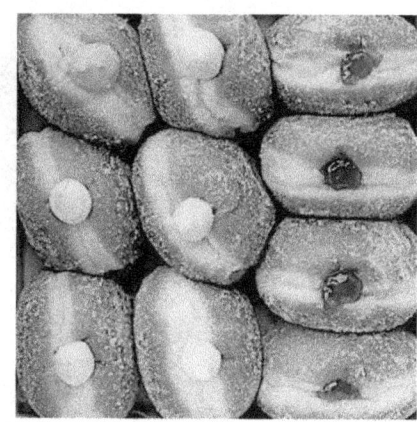

L

Leave donuts alone. In fact, it is expressly stated: "Do not; Do-Nots!" Donuts may surely be easy on the wallet - but they are also easy on killing many, yearly!

> *"Every chemically modified, chemically-induced food or snack is a novelty spot-kick you shouldn't want to take after turning thirty!"*
> – Sammy O. Joseph

#6: A Word of Caution on Red-meat.

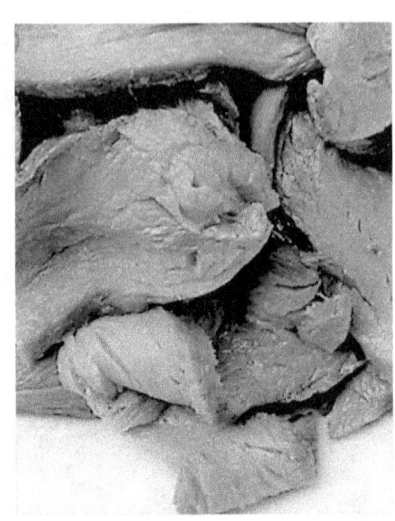

This is *not* venison. It is red meat. While occasional treat of venison may be *harmless*, red-meat – and its derivatives like minced beef, roast beef, meatball and corned beef, on the other hand, should be completely avoided the older you become! The same measure should be taken against pork and all its derivatives. (I wouldn't want to offend you, pork and sausage lovers, though!)

Avoid eating these meats as you age, for the sanctity of your long-term health. Anyone older than thirty years of age ought to substitute red-meat, pork and ribs – and their associates, with fish and healthy sea-foods!

#7: A Word of Caution on Processed food, Generally.

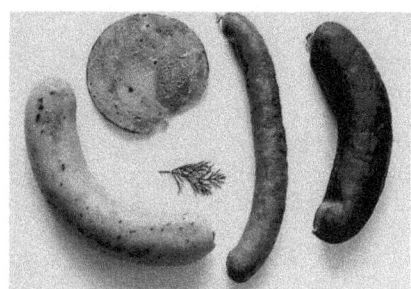

If you knew consuming processed foods will reduce your lifespan by a quarter of a hundred years, would you still eat them?

If on the other hand, you were told leading a certain lifestyle of exercise and physical engagement at the gym will increase your lifespan by a quarter of a century, would you choose to live or kill yourself early?

#8: Mental Awareness Needs.

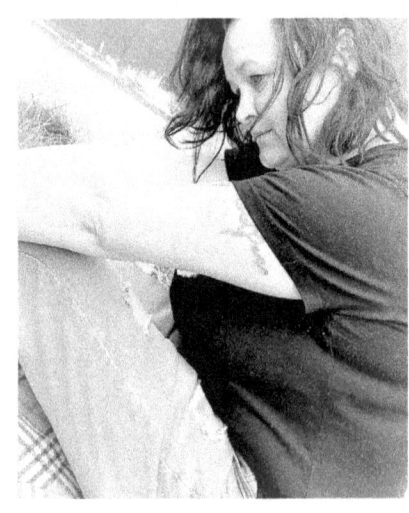

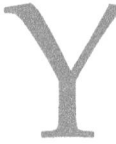

Your mental health awareness is as essential a need as the various other needs like physical, soulish, and spiritual awareness of your person!

One thing I learned as I grew older in the ministry of counseling and advice was the un-necessary stigma associated with just the mention of the phrase "mental illness." The truth is, one out of five, average, everyday people you meet on the street suffers from an undiagnosed mental fatigue or illness. According to Dr. Phillip C. McGraw, the popular American psychologist talk-show host *'Dr. Phil'*:

> *"20% of Americans – that is about 50 million people – suffer an undiagnosed mental illness yearly in the United States."*

Some Signs of Mental Illness

Some signs of undiagnosed mental illness include disinterest in observing a restful sleeping time at nights; waking up, and climbing out of bed! Dis-interest in getting ready for everyday living. Oversleep. The preference of a serenaded dark room to that floodlit by sunlight – and a general weakness of the mind. Other early signs of mental illness include erratic behaviors, treating living-companions to walking on eggshells around the house/office; inability to fully comprehend actions and their repercussions either in the short or the long run, a disoriented personality, delusion, a dishevelled, unkempt outlook, the belief in strange ideologies, uncontrolled anger outburst, shouting at the top of one's lungs above an average conversational tone, and the resultant epidemic of the opioid mess.

A majority of mental afflictions in the time of Christ Jesus – as is in our time – are as a result of demonic involvements in the lives of the sufferers. Or except through genetic transfer and of course, drug abuse! But as soon as Jesus, the Anointed One had rebuked and cast off those demons, every formerly possessed soul had immediately returned to a state of unperturbed tranquility and full mental health recovery!

Some Bizarre Behaviors Giving Unmissable Clues to Mental Unawareness

If you notice any of these behaviors in a loved one or someone you care about, it would be time to get to grips with them about their mental awareness needs. Many sufferers lack perception of themselves, suffer in silence, would rather dispute, argue – and possibly get violent with you in the process of your intervention plans.

Here are some abnormal functionalities of someone who may be in need of a mental health rescue – and my suggestion to you, is to handle the scenario with great caution and wisdom:

1.) Delusions, hallucinations or an extreme phobia that misconceives reflections off walls at night: (At dawn, what had kept the sufferer paralyzed with fear all-night-long could have been nothing but the shadow of a hung coat). If that were to be the case – particularly in a young child – you should hug them gently while holding them tightly, as to re-confirm to them of your protective care. Then find a re-assuring scriptural portion that re-enforces God's presence, to read to them. Portions of scripture like *Psalms 91, 23* and *46*.

2.) They pumped washing liquid onto the slug on the floor in order to get rid of it: If that were to be the case, refrain from shouting at them. Doing so may startle an already absent-mind. Lead them away from the scene of panic – and gently calm them down. You may eventually be both able to re-visit their actions – and also offer helpful suggestions.

3.) Sufferer practices more than appropriate soliloquy: Soliloquy is a serious, unhealthy absorption of self in self-talk, and engaging of oneself in solo conversation. (The one-million-dollar question remains: 'What is an appropriate soliloquy?')

Your answer to what an appropriate or inappropriate soliloquy is, would determine the appropriate medical, psychological or spiritual counseling you should seek.

4.) Lawn-mowing at 3 a.m: If that were to be the case, you should without engaging them in a disagreement, disengage the power-supply to the mower. Advise them how late into the night it was.

Let them know that it is against the law – socially acceptable behaviour – to disturb or disrupt the neighbhors' sleep.

You may need to be assertive with them as you intimate them with your urgent need to consult the hospital for an appointment with the General Practice Doctor, a Mental Health Practitioner, or a psychiatrist!

5.) *Loss of self-awareness:* Exhibiting personality disorders, compulsive lying, stealing, shoplifting, gambling away or spending huge sums of money on impulse. Anger outbursts, kicking holes into walls, issuing out punitive measures to pets; stepping into traffic as in jay-walking – and being general threats to oneself and others are all signs of heightened need for urgent, psychiatric diagnosis, evaluation and treatment!

Law enforcement teams and the Social Services teams of professionals should also, at this stage, be consulted!

6.) *Unwillingness to get a paying job – and/or the inability to hold down a job*: If any should not work, Scripture says they should not eat | 2 Thessalonians 3:10. It's that simple. They should not eat and they should not be encouraged with continued stipends or pocket monies, in case they were grown teens. It is called: "Tough love!"

7.) *Prone to instigate an assault, physical altercations coupled with an abundance of foul language:* (I would advise the same course of action as enumerated in point number (5) above).

8.) Over-medicating – and overdosing on prescription drugs; dealing in illegal drugs and narcotics, supplying drugs – and harboring drug users: Self-medicating and the abuse of either prescriptive medicines or drugs is against the law of the land. Law enforcement teams must be notified of such acts.

9.) Experimenting with – and getting hooked on LSD, acid, weed, cocaine, amphetamine that causes uncontrollable shaking, convulsion and turning blue; and

10.) Exhibitions of bipolar disorder, schizophrenia, ADHD, ADD, extreme OCD, Bulimia, binge-eating – and other disorders!

I have deliberately arranged these signs or manifestations of abnormal mental health issues in an upscale fashion; from the least worrying to the most troubling, in *"Scales 1 - 10"*

As you can see, anything above Scale 3 must, as a point of strict observation, be reported to the right professionals!

Please demonstrate love to your loved ones. There should be no shame and stigma attached to anyone suffering from mental illness, as there's no shaming anyone undergoing treatments to battle, say another dreaded, killer disease, as cancer!

#9: 'Gymnos' Acknowledgment.

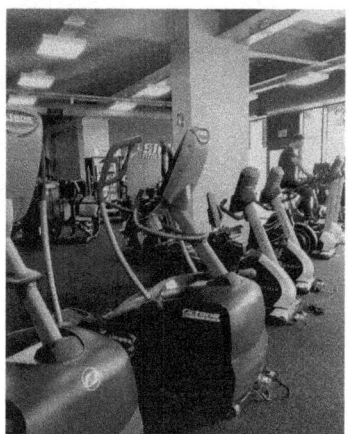

The word *"gymnos"* is derived from the ancient Greek term meaning "naked." I would for the sake of our discussion here borrow and apply that word to our everyday vocabulary and terminology, regarding mental health issues.

Please, for the sake of the love of God, if you notice that the behavioral inclinations of any of your loved ones are becoming bizarre or suspicious, please kindly show some empathy, care – and become 'naked' with them about those issues?

You owe them a sense of *"gymnos"* to lovingly confront them with the proofs of their bizarreness! Mental illness, as earlier said on the preceding pages, is no different from any other disease or ailment! The society of responsive, compassionate souls ought to be butt-naked truthful with reality in approaching mental awareness needs and the issues surrounding the preventative treatment of both psychological and spiritual maladies!

#10: The Appropriate Use of a Gymnasium – Or other Health & Fitness Facilities.

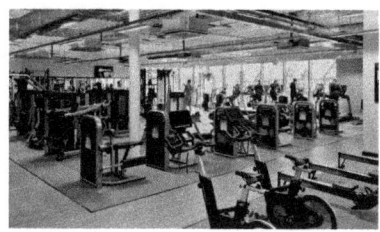

I

It is an undoubted truth: Daily exercise routines would give you a bumper-harvest yield of anything from between a score and a quarter of a century added years to your longevity. More, the appropriate use of the facilities in a gymnasium will de-stress and keep you healthier. Exercises such as running on a treadmill, rowing, cycling, lifting weights, CrossFit-training, swimming and so on will boost your overall health pattern, mentally, emotionally and physically.

Whatever activities you can engage in outside of the gymnasium too will become added advantage to your general health and well-being, even as you advance in age! Please do *not* let go of your body, mind, and spirit. Be a total-person.

PART TEN

A Closing Remark

10
A Closing Remark

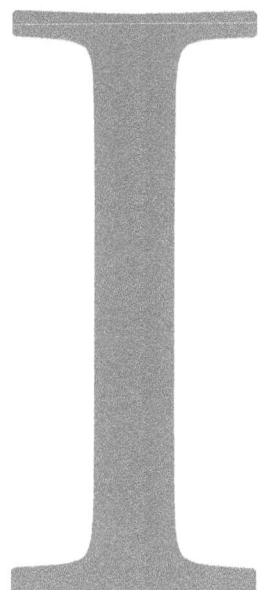

I hope you have been blessed through this book. If my lessons have in any way enriched your life, please kindly send me a note today, write me a review, or find me on most social media platforms. You may also e-mail or simply text me to *(+44) 7758-195466*. My contact addresses are at the back of the book.

Be a blessing. Purchase copies of this book for your family members and friends! Help celebrate the news of my half-centenary existence on this planet – and by thus doing, support the advancement of the Kingdom of our God!

God's peace be multiplied unto you as you too grow in grace. Amen

Sincerely,

Sammy Joseph.

Visit Us if You're in our City

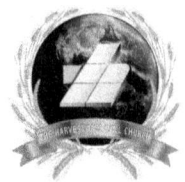

The Harvestways Int'l Church
(Birmingham, U.K.)
Holloway Hall
Northfield, Birmingham,
England, United Kingdom
B31 1TT
Sunday Worship: 12 noon
Wednesday Bible Study: 8pm
Home Cell Friday Prayer Meeting: 7pm
Tel: (+44) 7758195466
e-mail: admin@harvestways.org

The Harvestways Int'l Church
(Nigeria, West Africa)
1 & 2 Harvest Way, Off Elewura Street
Behind Zartech / GLO Office,
Off Elewura Street
Challenge, Ibadan, Oyo State,
Nigeria, West Africa.
Sunday Worship: 9am
Tuesday Bible Study: 6pm
e-mail: nigeria@harvestways.org

Other Books by the Author

Other books by the author are available at any Christian bookshop near you; or from our website: *harvestways.org*

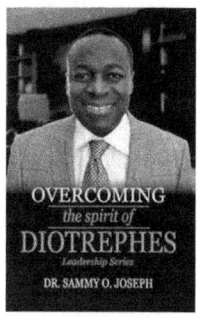

Overcoming the spirit of DIOTREPHES
(Leadership Series)
Whether you're a follower or a leader — particularly a Christian leader, this is a book you would love to read! *"I know you must have met or crossed paths — at a time or another, with a character the like of Diotrephes who had occupied a high seat of power and influence. But you had never actually been able to put a finger on the reason(s) why such a so-called, 'born-again', child of God could have acted so fleshly: Their bizarreness had left you in quite, a state of shock! Well, this book has detailed all you needed to overcome the spirit of Diotrephes"*, writes Dr. Joseph

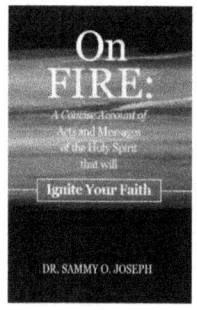

On Fire *(Leadership Series)*
"After Dr. Taylor had prayed, the Lord had given me a flashing vision: I had seen Miela arise from that same bed — and taken two strong steps in total health — before bursting into a run! Oh, by the gift of interpretation of dreams and visions, I knew the symbolism of that vision; so I had prophesied accordingly, by the same Holy Spirit …"
Thus opens the *On FIRE* with this vivid, poignant, true story of triumphant healing that serves as the curtain-raiser for many more of its kind beautifully told throughout the book. (*214 pages*).

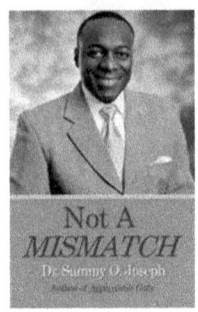

Not A Mismatch
Affixing labels, numbers and digits on objects may not be inherently wrong, generally speaking; but when they have been employed for derogatory purposes, I may have to become the very first to confidently shoot my right hand up into the air, well above my head and demand logical explanations as to why that should be! My message to you, therefore, is very simple: Your adverse life experiences or circumstances do not make you irrelevant. No matter your background, color, ethnicity or creed, the Creator has your very name written in the palms of His hands – and calls you by that name. You are not a misfit (*168 pages*).

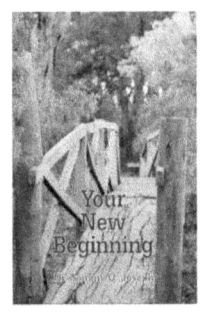

Your New Beginning
A new beginning doesn't just show up. Success doesn't just arrive on anybody's laps; it only will arrive as a result of a deliberate, changed mindset. In this piece, the author makes the receptivity of the Word of God the catalyst to the change that births your desired new beginning. Says he: *"Whenever or wherever occurs the reception of the words of the Lord into a human spirit, there is illumination ... And not only illumination but warmth, glow, radiance, heat and the fire that purges! Thirsty for the Change; Hunger for the World!"*

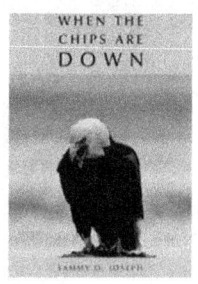

When the Chips Are DOWN

You will be enraptured by the way the author has deployed sheer literary genus and a sharp, enrapturing writing style to describe the intuitive bald eagle — how he triumphs over his gruesome moulting season in the wild. Learn in this book, your very personalized "way of escape" provided by the loving Heavenly Father out of the feelings of despair, despondency, desolation and depression. (*110 pages*)

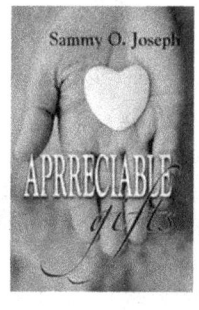

APPRECIABLE Gifts

Seekers in quest of attaining inner peace with the heavenly Father, deepening satisfaction in their friendships/relationships, healings from life's brokenness — enhancing their sexuality and marriages need search no further. Within the pages of *Appreciable Gifts* lie your missing trophies! Irrespective of your status in life, if your heart desires to learn the most essential tips on how to 'spruce up' your 3-D relationships: vertical, horizontal and downwards, *'Appreciable Gifts'* will show you how! (*183 pages*)

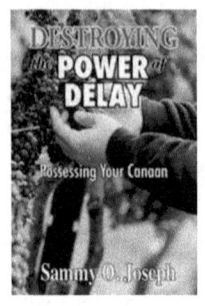

DESTROYING the Power of DELAY
This book is an expository piece of work, written in a scriptural, thought-provoking style. The author aimed at sharing with you from the experiences gathered over more than two decades of counselling in ministry, how to avoid the endearing long arms of delay; and if you're already entangled in a wild romance with the hated alien, the quickest way of escape from him. Real-life issues such as *'Causes of Delay', 'Who Should Care for the Elderly?', 'Wisdom Handling Inextricable Covenant Relationships', 'Liberating Financial Management and Dealing with Indebtedness'* are adequately discussed. Others topics include: *'How to Effectively Handle Mid-life Crisis, Depression, Barrenness.'* (*220 pages*)

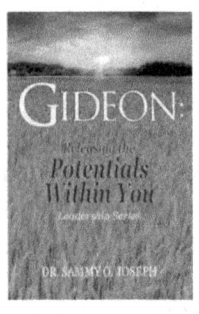

GIDEON: Releasing the Potentials Within You (Leadership Series)
This book draws analogies from the life of Gideon (one of Israel's Judges) and applies them to how you can effectively release the hidden potentials within you. Written in easy, straightforward, simple language, you will find basic practical insights that will help lift you above common mediocrity levels in life (*176 pages*).

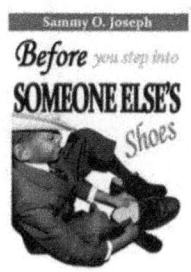

Before You Step into Someone Else's Shoes
This book contains *easy-to-do* guides on how you will not repeat the costly mistakes made by others faced with a fresh opportunity to begin anew after suffering a heavy setback. We have also provided essential checklists to anyone willing to *step into shoes* ordained of God for them — as well as checkmating the mutineers! (*46 pages*)

Become a *Sammy Joseph Ministries* Vision Partner

Our commitment is to:
- *Pray — and cover you daily in prayers, that God's undeniable blessings be upon your you and your household;*
- *Keep ministering the Word of God diligently;*
- *Minister to you once a month via a telephone call from us;*
- *Minister to you in a personal newsletter from Dr. Sammy Joseph — at least quarterly;*
- *Issue you an official partner certificate; and,*
- *Offer you from time to time, special, discounted gifts for your spiritual growth and upliftment through our website, programs and outreaches.*

Your commitment is to:
- *Pray for us always;*
- *Be committed to support our broadcasts, meetings and outreaches in your area;*
- *Support us financially with your monthly 'seed' as said in Philippians 4:17; and,*
- *Always speak positive words of affirmation on the ministry, Dr. Joseph — and his family.*

If you would love to:
- *Become a vision partner / supporter of Sammy Joseph Ministries;*
- *Become a volunteer at any of our outreaches;*
- *Invite Dr. Joseph to minister for you in your church, train your ministers / staff; or*

- *Help organize the three day International Experience Harvestways Conference in your church, city or country.*

Please write to:
Sammy Joseph Ministries
Holloway Hall,
P.O. Box 15129
Birmingham, England, B45 5DJ
admin@harvestways.org
Call: (+44) 775-8195466 / 121-258-2299

THANK YOU!

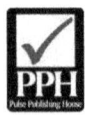

Contact Addresses
United Kingdom, Europe
Pulse Publishing House
Sammy Joseph Ministries
Holloway Hall,
Box 15129
Birmingham, England
West Midlands, U.K
B45 5DJ
Mobile: *(+44) 7758195466*

pulsepublishinghouse@harvestways.org

Nigeria, Africa
Pulse Publishing House
Plots 1 & 2, Harvest Way, Off Elewura Street
Behind Zartech / GLO Office,
Challenge, Ibadan,
Nigeria, West Africa.

pulsepublishinghouse@harvestways.org

PULSE Publishing House also avails you a secure processing and prompt worldwide shipment if you order from.harvestways.org

If you would also love to become a distributor; contact us, today!

All our books and products are sold online wherever books are sold, including Barnesandnoble.com & Amazon.com

www.ingramcontent.com/pod-product-compliance
Lightning Source LLC
LaVergne TN
LVHW041619070426
835507LV00008B/332